Vitamin C Fortification of Food Aid Commodities

Final Report

Committee on International Nutrition—
Vitamin C in Food Aid Commodities

Food and Nutrition Board
Board on International Health

INSTITUTE OF MEDICINE

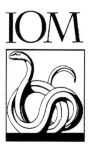

IOM

NATIONAL ACADEMY PRESS
Washington, D.C. 1997

NATIONAL ACADEMY PRESS • 2101 Constitution Avenue, N.W. • Washington, DC 20418

NOTICE: The project that is the subject of this report was approved by the Governing Board of the National Research Council, whose members are drawn from the councils of the National Academy of Sciences, the National Academy of Engineering, and the Institute of Medicine. The members of the committee responsible for the report were chosen for their special competences and with regard for appropriate balance.

This report has been reviewed by a group other than the authors according to procedures approved by a Report Review Committee consisting of members of the National Academy of Sciences, the National Academy of Engineering, and the Institute of Medicine.

The Institute of Medicine was chartered in 1970 by the National Academy of Sciences to enlist distinguished members of the appropriate professions in the examination of policy matters pertaining to the health of the public. In this, the Institute acts under the Academy's 1863 congressional charter responsibility to be an adviser to the federal government and its own initiative in identifying issues of medical care, research, and education. Dr. Kenneth I. Shine is president of the Institute of Medicine.

Support for this project was provided by the Office of Health and Nutrition, United States Agency for International Development, Cooperative Agreement No. DPE-5951-A-00-0035-00. The opinions expressed in this report are those of the Committee on International Nutrition and do not necessarily reflect the views of the sponsor.

International Standard Book No. 0-309-05999-2

Additional copies of *Vitamin C Fortification of Food Aid Commodities: Final Report* are available for sale from the National Academy Press, 2101 Constitution Avenue, N.W., Box 285, Washington, DC 20055. Call (800) 624-6242 or (202) 334-3313 (in the Washington metropolitan area) or visit the NAP's on-line bookstore at **www.nap.edu**.

For more information about the Institute of Medicine, visit the IOM home page at **www2.nas.edu/iom**.

Printed in the United States of America.

The serpent has been a symbol of long life, healing, and knowledge among almost all cultures and religions since the beginning of recorded history. The image adopted as a logotype by the Institute of Medicine is based on a relief carving from ancient Greece, now held by the Staatliche Museen in Berlin.

Preface

Over the past 5 years, there has been considerable interest and focus on micronutrient fortification of rations provided in international food relief programs. The United States makes significant contributions to food aid authorized by Public Law (P.L.) 480, Title II as the Food for Peace Program. This program is administered by the U.S. Agency for International Development's Bureau of Humanitarian Response (BHR).

Beginning in fiscal year 1993, congressional appropriations committees urged the U.S. Agency for International Development (USAID) to more than double the amount of vitamin C added to blended commodities exported through P.L. 480, Title II programs (Foreign Operations, Export Financing, and Related Programs Appropriations Bill, 1993, S. Rpt. 102-419; 1994, S. Rpt. 103-142) (see Appendix A). The commodities that were targeted for increased fortification were corn–soy blend (CSB) and wheat–soy blend (WSB)—the only commodities that are fortified with vitamin C. These blended foods are also fortified with an array of other vitamins and minerals and require minimal cooking. The stated purpose of the increased vitamin C fortification of these blended foods was to improve the health of food aid recipients and reduce the need for, and cost of, later medical interventions (Foreign Operations, Export Financing, and Related Programs Appropriations Bill, 1994, S. Rpt. 103-142). Supplemental rations of these highly fortified, blended foods are provided to refugees and displaced persons in camps and to beneficiaries of development feeding programs that are targeted largely toward mothers and children. The 1995 congressional appropriations conference report asked for information on the cost of increased fortification and the stability of vitamin C throughout the shipping process (Making Appropriations for the Foreign Operations, Export Financing, and Related Programs for the fiscal year ending September 30, 1995, Conference Report, 1995, H. Rpt. 103-633).

The stability of vitamin C (L-ascorbic acid) is of concern because this is the most labile vitamin in foods. Its main loss during processing and storage is from oxidation, which is accelerated by light, oxygen, heat, increased pH, high moisture content (water activity), and the presence of copper or ferrous salts. Oxidative losses also occur during food preparation, and additional vitamin C may be lost if it dissolves into cooking liquid that is then discarded.

In 1995, the Senate Appropriations Committee Report 104-143, "Foreign Operations, Export Financing, and Related Programs Appropriation Bill, 1996," directed USAID to initiate a pilot program to increase the vitamin C content of CSB and WSB to 90 mg/100 g and to report on the results (Appendix A). In response, USAID set up a cooperative agreement with the organization SUSTAIN (Sharing United States Technology to Aid in the Improvement of Nutrition) to devise and implement the pilot program. USAID also asked the Institute of Medicine(IOM) to form a committee to address the cost-effectiveness and advisability of increasing the level of vitamin C used to fortify the food aid commodities CSB and WSB. The Committee on International Nutrition—Vitamin C in Food Aid Commodities was constituted in response to this request.

The committee's overall task was to address the cost-effectiveness and advisability of scaling up Title II commodity vitamin C fortification to improve recipients' diet, nutrition, and health. The committee's initial report, *Vitamin C in Food Aid Commodities: Initial Review of a Pilot Program* (IOM, 1996), addressed the first part of its specific tasks. In particular, it reviewed the pilot program designed by SUSTAIN, presented recommendations for its improvement, and identified additional types of information needed to complete the overall task. The committee emphasized the potential value of collecting data from emergency feeding programs, as well as from development programs, and of collecting samples on-site to determine vitamin C losses during food preparation. It requested additional data on cost, and on the prevalence of scurvy and insufficient vitamin C and iron intakes in populations that receive blended foods.

SUSTAIN had access to the IOM's initial report as it completed its pilot program. SUSTAIN and USAID presented *Results Report on the Vitamin C Pilot Program* (Ranum and Chomé, 1997) to the Committee on International Nutrition shortly before the committee's second meeting. That report covers the following topics: the uniformity of vitamin C distribution in WSB and CSB at five plant sites; the stability of vitamin C from point of production to distribution in both CSB shipped to India and WSB shipped to Haiti; the variation of vitamin C distribution within bags after shipping and handling; cooking methods and the retention of vitamin C following food preparation by recipients; and estimates of the cost of increasing vitamin C fortification from 40 to 90 mg/100 g. The report also provided responses to each of the special information requests submitted by the Committee on International Nutrition.

In the present report the committee reviews and evaluates the final report of the pilot program, determines the cost-effectiveness of scaling up vitamin C fortification, makes recommendations concerning the advisability of increasing vitamin C fortification, and discusses alternative mechanisms for providing vitamin C to refugee populations at risk for vitamin C deficiency. The committee also identifies areas in which additional research is needed to more effectively meet nutritional needs in emergency feeding situations.

The chair and the entire committee would like to express their sincere appreciation to the representatives of SUSTAIN, the U.S. Department of Agriculture, and USAID who met with the committee to answer questions about data in the SUSTAIN preliminary and final reports and provided additional information to the committee as it became available. The committee also thanks Judit Katona-Apte of the United Nations' World Food Programme, who provided information on emergency feeding programs. The committee expresses its gratitude for the staff assistance and support provided by the IOM. We are indebted to Carol Suitor, who served as study director for the initial committee report; Mary Poos, study director for the committee's final report; Diane Johnson and Geraldine Kennedo, senior project assistants; Mike Edington, managing editor; Claudia Carl, administrative associate for report review; and Carlos Gabriel, financial associate. The committee especially thanks Allison Yates, director of the Food and Nutrition Board; Karen Hein, executive officer; and Kenneth I. Shine, president of the Institute of Medicine. The work of the committee was made possible only by the contributions and support of these individuals.

> Lindsay H. Allen, *Chair*
> Committee on International Nutrition—
> Vitamin C in Food Aid Commodities

Contents

EXECUTIVE SUMMARY   1
  Background and Charge to the Committee, 2
  Methods, 3
  Conclusions, 3
  Recommendations, 5
  Research Recommendations, 6

1 INTRODUCTION   9
  The Committee's Task, 13
  The Study Process, 14

2 VITAMIN C: NEEDS AND FUNCTIONS   17
  Prevalence of Scurvy, 18
  Vitamin C Requirements, 20
  Other Functions of Vitamin C, 21
  Vitamin C and Iron Absorption, 21

3 COST-EFFECTIVENESS ANALYSIS   23
  Effectiveness, 23
  Cost, 26
  Cost-Effectiveness Estimate, 27

4 RESULTS OF THE VITAMIN C PILOT PROGRAM   37
  Summary of the Pilot Program, 37
  Major Findings of the Pilot Program, 41

5 CRITIQUE OF THE PILOT PROGRAM   47
  Uniformity of Blended Commodities, 47

    Capability of the Production Process to Meet Product
        Specifications, 48
    Stability of Vitamin C During Transport and Storage, 49
    Vitamin C Cooking Losses, 50

6   **CONCLUSIONS AND RECOMMENDATIONS**   53
    Conclusions, 53
    Recommendations, 58

REFERENCES   63

APPENDIXES
A   Legislative Language for Increased Vitamin C Fortification, 67
B   SUSTAIN Report Executive Summary, 73
C   Letter from the United Nations World Food Programme, 81
D   Biographical Sketches, 85

LIST OF TABLES AND BOXES

Tables

1-1 Ingredient Composition of Corn–Soy Blend (CSB) and Wheat–Soy Blend
     (WSB), 10
1-2 Selected Nutrient Composition of Corn–Soy Blend (CSB), 10
1-3 Selected Nutrient Composition of Wheat–Soy Blend (WSB), 11
3-1 Possible Consequences of Added Cost from Higher Vitamin C Levels, 28
4-1 Summary of Vitamin C Retention After Cooking, 41
4-2 Tanzania Samples—CSB Food Preparations, Vitamin C Data, 43
4-3 Haiti Samples—WSB Food Preparations, Vitamin C Data, 45
5-1 Summary of Food Preparation Samples Collected in Selected
     Countries, 50

Boxes

4-1 Schedule of the CSB Special Procurement from Production
     to Distribution in the Refugee Camps of Western Tanzania, 40
4-2 Schedule of the WSB Special Procurement from Production to Distribution
     in Haiti, 40

Executive Summary

It is estimated that the requirement worldwide for grain, simply to maintain current food consumption and meet emergency needs, will double in the next decade. In some regions, most notably sub-Saharan Africa and South Asia, the stagnation of nutritional improvement combined with a rapid rise in population has resulted in an actual increase in the total number of malnourished children. Most of sub-Saharan Africa is now worse off nutritionally than 10 years ago. Globally, nearly 200 million children under 5 years of age continue to be malnourished. At the same time, global food aid deliveries have declined continuously since 1993.

The United States contributes a variety of food commodities to global food aid through the Food for Peace Program authorized by Public Law (P.L.) 480, Title II and administered by the U.S. Agency for International Development (USAID). These commodities include cereal grains (corn, wheat, rice, sorghum), pulses (peas, bean, lentils), vegetable oils, and a variety of milled cereal and blended products (e.g., wheat flour, corn meal, soy flour). In 1996, approximately 1.7 million metric tons (MT) of food aid commodities valued at more than $840 million were distributed through Title II programs.

In addition to general protein-energy malnutrition (PEM), international food relief organizations are focusing increased attention on the global incidence of micronutrient deficiencies. Deficiencies of vitamin A, iron, and iodine are widespread in developing countries. Deficiencies of micronutrients such as vitamin C, niacin, and thiamin have occurred in localized areas, primarily in Africa and South Asia. To address some of these micronutrient deficiencies, two blended, fortified commodities are produced for distribution in the Food for Peace Program, corn–soy blend (CSB) and wheat–soy blend (WSB). These blended foods consist of a mixture of the appropriate cereal

1

(gelatinized cornmeal or wheat flour and wheat protein concentrate), defatted soy flour, and soybean oil; they are fortified with 6 essential minerals and 11 vitamins, including vitamin C. These foods are provided as ration supplements to refugees and internally displaced persons in camps and to recipients of development aid programs that are targeted largely towards mothers and children. The United States supplied 84 percent of the total fortified, blended foods used worldwide in 1996.

The current level of vitamin C fortification of CSB and WSB (40 mg/100 g) is based on the 1974 National Research Council (NRC) recommendations for children up to 11 years of age, by assuming an intake of 100 g of blended cereal per day. However, the Food and Agriculture Organization (FAO) and the World Health Organization (WHO) recommend a minimal requirement of 20 mg of vitamin C per day for children up to 5 years of age and 30 mg for adults; the United Nations High Commissioner on Refugees (UNHCR) recommends 27 mg of vitamin C per day.

BACKGROUND AND CHARGE TO THE COMMITTEE

Beginning in fiscal year (FY) 1993, U.S. congressional appropriations committees urged USAID to increase the amount of vitamin C added to CSB and WSB from 40 mg/100 g of cereal blend to 90–100 mg/100g of cereal blend. The stated purpose of the increased vitamin C fortification of these blended foods was to improve the health of food aid recipients, particularly new mothers and infants, and to reduce the need for, and cost of, later medical interventions. An initial study commissioned by USAID on various options for appropriate micronutrient fortification recommended that vitamin C fortification not be increased until additional information was obtained on the stability of vitamin C during transport, storage, and preparation. The FY 1996 Senate Appropriations Committee directed USAID to initiate a pilot program to increase the vitamin C content of CSB and WSB to 90 mg/100 g and to report the results. In response, USAID initiated a cooperative agreement with the organization SUSTAIN (Sharing United States Technology to Aid in the Improvement of Nutrition) to devise and implement the pilot program. USAID also requested that the Institute of Medicine (IOM) address the cost-effectiveness and advisability of scaling up vitamin C fortification of these blended food aid commodities to improve recipients' diet, nutrition, and health. The Committee on International Nutrition—Vitamin C in Food Aid Commodities of the Food and Nutrition Board was constituted in response to this request.

The committee was charged with review of the proposed pilot program, examining it for soundness of scientific and technical design in relation to (1) monitoring the presence and stability of vitamin C in food aid commodities and (2) assessing the dietary intake of vitamin C, nutritional status, and health status of recipients. Based on this review, the committee prepared a brief report *Vitamin C in Food Aid Commodities: Initial Review of a Pilot Program* (IOM,

1996). For the present report, the committee's specific charge was to assess the results of the pilot program; determine the advisability of increasing vitamin C fortification to improve recipients' diet, nutrition, and health; and determine the cost-effectiveness of increased vitamin C fortification of food aid commodities compared with other means of delivering vitamin C.

METHODS

The committee met twice during the study. At the first meeting, an open session was held with representatives from USAID, SUSTAIN, the U.S. Department of Agriculture, the Food and Drug Administration, the Kellogg Corporation, and Protein Grain Products International. The committee reviewed SUSTAIN's proposed pilot program and prepared a preliminary report. Committee staff conducted an extensive literature search to attain a more global view of the reported incidence of scurvy in refugee populations, the effects of vitamin C on iron absorption, and other potential health effects of vitamin C supplementation. At the second meeting, the committee reviewed SUSTAIN's final report of the results of the pilot program, conducted a videoconference with USAID and SUSTAIN representatives, and teleconferenced with a representative of the United Nations' World Food Programme for further insights into global food aid needs. Additional information was obtained on the tonnage of CSB and WSB produced, their distribution in development versus emergency relief programs, and cost information on various methods of providing vitamin C. These activities provided the committee with the information on which it based its deliberations.

CONCLUSIONS

Dietary deficiency of vitamin C eventually leads to scurvy. Clinical signs of scurvy include swollen or bleeding gums, petechial hemorrhages, joint pain and swelling, and follicular hyperkeratosis. These symptoms are associated with plasma (or serum) vitamin C values of less than 0.2 mg/dl. Minimum dietary levels ranging from 6.5 to 10 mg per day have been reported necessary to prevent clinical signs of scurvy. These same levels have been found to produce marked improvement of mild clinical signs of scurvy; however, higher doses (32 mg up to 600 mg per day) were needed for more rapid improvement of symptoms and saturation of body stores.

Scurvy outbreaks have occurred among refugee populations entirely dependent on emergency relief rations that provide less than 2 mg of vitamin C per day per person. The greatest number of outbreaks occurred in the 1980s in Somalia. Except for a recurring mild scurvy outbreak among Bhutanese refugees in Nepal, all other outbreaks in the past two decades have been in refugee camps in the greater Horn of Africa (Ethiopia, Kenya, Somalia, Sudan). The reason for this localized occurrence is not clear, but it may be due to the location of these camps in isolated areas away from local populations and markets and on land unsuitable for cultivation. Thus, the need for higher vitamin C fortification of CSB or WSB would be sporadic and localized.

Only a small proportion (7 percent) of U.S.-supplied CSB and WSB is designated for emergency feeding programs in East Africa, where scurvy has been reported. Thus, fully 93 percent of the cost of adding more vitamin C to blended, fortified foods as a strategy for preventing scurvy would be wasted. If a fixed dollar amount is assumed available for the purchase of food aid commodities, increasing the vitamin C content to 90 mg/100 g—at an estimated increased cost of $6.33/metric tons (MT)—would lead to forgoing the provision of fortified blended commodities as a supplement (30 g per person per day) in emergency food aid to approximately 425,800 recipients. This situation is not conducive to improving their nutrition and health status. Alternative approaches for the prevention of scurvy should be explored where the availability of locally produced vitamin C-rich foods is low.

Furthermore, results of SUSTAIN's pilot program identified unacceptable variability in the fortification levels of vitamin C in CSB, which raises serious questions about the ability of manufacturers to meet specified nutrient levels in the final product. None of the four CSB plants sampled consistently achieved target fortification levels, and two of them were outside specifications almost 60 percent of the time. Given the pervasive problem of lack of uniformity, the committee believes it would be inappropriate to increase any micronutrient fortification of these commodities without better manufacturing controls.

Information from the pilot study indicates that vitamin C losses during shipping and storage are not a concern, but losses of vitamin C during cooking may be a major limiting factor, ranging from a low of 52 percent up to as much as 82 percent lost. However, data for vitamin C losses during cooking were not conclusive because of a number of variables introduced, particularly the variability of vitamin C concentration in the starting blends and the very limited number of samples analyzed.

In addition, although iron deficiency appears to be a much more widespread problem than scurvy in emergency feeding situations, the use of higher levels of vitamin C fortification to enhance iron absorption is not a cost-effective method of improving iron status. Even if the current cost of fortifying blended foods with iron ($1.61/MT) could be cut in half, the net effect of improving iron absorption through the addition of vitamin C would still be a cost increase of $5.52/MT.

RECOMMENDATIONS

1. The level of vitamin C fortification of blended food aid commodities should *NOT* be increased to 90 mg/100 g, but should be maintained at the current level of 40 mg/100 g. Based on the reported incidence of scurvy and the quantity of U.S.-supplied blended food commodities going to regions where scurvy has been reported, increasing vitamin C fortification of all CSB and WSB is not cost-effective.

2. Strengthen health surveillance systems in refugee camps to monitor population risks of vitamin C deficiency and scurvy and to initiate a timely response. Risk factors for vitamin C deficiency and scurvy should be monitored at the community and/or camp level. Some risk factors that have been identified as potentially useful for such monitoring include populations totally dependent on food aid (e.g., displaced and famine-affected populations); duration of stay in a refugee camp; seasonality: dry season and inability to cultivate; market failure, limited local supplies of fresh produce, or lack of resources to trade for other food sources; poor acceptance of donated foods, especially the blended, fortified foods, resulting from cultural preferences; and difficult access by relief organizations because of war or remoteness. At the individual level, risk factors include age and physiological status (young children, pregnant and lactating women, and the elderly have been found more susceptible).

3. Target identified populations at risk for scurvy with appropriate vitamin C interventions. There are several possible strategies to achieve increased vitamin C supplementation: (1) increased access to local foods and markets; (2) local fortification of commodities in the country or region where the emergency is occurring, as is currently practiced in some regions; and (3) use of vitamin C tablets if scurvy is already present. Alternatively, an increased total daily ration of conventionally fortified, blended food would be appropriate to an emergency feeding situation and would increase the intake of other important nutrients such as energy, protein, and iron, as well as vitamin C. Another possibility might be for USAID's Bureau of Humanitarian Response to investigate the logistics of managing two supplies of CSB and/or WSB, the conventionally fortified blends and a small proportion of highly fortified blends that would be targeted as part of the general ration only to situations where the risk of vitamin C deficiency is high and continues for several months.

4. Improve the uniformity of blended food aid commodities by implementing specific product and process procedures. Delivery of vitamin and mineral fortification via food aid commodities to target populations depends on the manufacturing facilities' ability to comply with formulation and finished product specifications. To improve the uniformity of blended food, the following remedial initiatives are recommended:

• Formulation document—a formal reporting of the formulation and ingredients used to generate a particular product or blend.

• Product specifications—instituting procedures for analytical quality control to monitor compliance with fortification levels defined by product specification. Inability of manufacturer to comply can result in loss of contract.

• Methods and sampling procedures—listing of all statistical process control procedures, analytical procedures, test methods, and appropriate sampling protocols.

• Operating guide—a formal document that provides a blueprint for operating a process. It includes a process description for each step, a review of normal operating conditions, control actions (the set of steps necessary to maintain a quality operation), and a discussion of the impact of each process step on product quality.

• Control plan—a master document that keeps track of a plant's record keeping. It lists the specification or test to be performed, the source of the authority for the test, who is responsible for conducting the test, the test frequency, where the test is recorded, what action to take, and where to file or who must receive the report.

• HACCP (Hazards Analysis Critical Control Points) plan—a preventive system to identify key areas of process control to avoid food safety risks.

Measurements of improvement include analytical sampling and analysis of key fortification nutrients, regular audits of plant performance, maintenance of calibration records for all metering equipment, and maintenance of usage records for all vitamin and mineral premixes.

RESEARCH RECOMMENDATIONS

The committee has identified several areas in which additional research would be most helpful in alleviating potential vitamin C deficiencies and evaluating the appropriateness of any overall vitamin C fortification of U.S. commodities.

1. Research the epidemiology of vitamin C deficiencies. Ascertain the incidence of scurvy in displaced populations and analyze this according to the amount of blended, fortified foods received. The incidence of scurvy among those receiving blended foods at currently prescribed levels will permit assessment of the need to increase fortification or seek alternative approaches. Develop and validate predictors of populations at risk of vitamin C deficiency among refugees so as to institute local fortification.

2. Research and develop means to increase consumption of local foods rich in vitamin C. This may also be achieved by purchasing these foods for refugees, but it may be done more cost-effectively by decreasing barriers to barter and trade in refugee camps.

3. Research and evaluate appropriate ration sizes of blended foods. More information is needed on the amounts of blended foods distributed to those at risk for scurvy in displaced populations. Currently, no good information is available on actual quantities distributed. This may also indicate that much higher levels of fortification than are currently being considered would be necessary for those at most risk because they could be receiving smaller rations.

4. Research and evaluate methods for campsite vitamin C fortification. This would be the most cost-effective approach to fortification because the need is rare and the cost of vitamin C is relatively high.

5. Research alternative forms of vitamin C available for fortification. The limited data available on cooking losses when using the current ethyl cellulose-coated product indicate a need to develop other vitamin C products that are more stable to heating in dilute solutions.

1

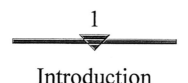

Introduction

The United States contributes a variety of food commodities to global food aid through the Food for Peace Program authorized by Public Law (P.L.) 480, Title II. These commodities include cereal grains (corn, wheat, rice, sorghum), pulses (peas, beans, lentils), and a variety of milled cereal and blended products (e.g., wheat flour, bulgur, cornmeal, soy flour, soy flour–cornmeal blend). These commodities are procured for the U.S. Agency for International Development (USAID) by the U.S. Department of Agriculture (USDA)/Export Operations Division/Farm Service Agency. The Commodity Credit Corporation of USDA develops specifications and issues invitations to bid on supplying commodities for the export program. The commodities are produced by commercial companies in the United States under inspection by the USDA Federal Grain Inspection Service. P.L. 480 imposes a variety of restrictions: for example, all ingredients must have been produced and mixed in the United States, and the supplier must deliver the commodity dockside for ship transport. In 1996, approximately 1.7 million metric tons of food aid commodities valued at more than $840 million were distributed through Title II programs (USAID, 1996).

Two blended, fortified commodities are produced for distribution in the Food for Peace Program: corn–soy blend (CSB) and wheat–soy blend (WSB). These blended foods are a mixture of the appropriate cereal (gelatinized cornmeal or wheat flour and wheat protein concentrate), defatted soy flour, and soybean oil; they are fortified with 6 essential minerals and 11 vitamins (Table 1-1). The blended product has a higher protein (20 percent for WSB, 16–17 percent for CSB) and energy content (360 kcal/100 g for WSB, 380 kcal/100 g for CSB) than unblended cereal commodities as well as higher levels of vitamins and minerals due to fortification (Tables 1-2 and 1-3).

TABLE 1-1. Ingredient Composition of Corn–Soy Blend (CSB) and Wheat–Soy Blend (WSB)

Ingredient	CSB	WSB
Corn Meal (processed,gelatinzed)	69.8%	—
Wheat Fractions, Total[a]	—	73.1%
Soy Flour (defatted, toasted)	21.9%	20.0%
Soy Bean Oil (stabilized)	5.5%	4.0%
Mineral Premix[b]	2.7%	2.8%
Vitamin Premix[c]	0.1%	0.1%

[a] Wheat fraction may consist of 53.1 percent bulgur and 20 percent wheat protein concentrate (enzyme inactivated), or 38.1 percent wheat flour (cooked) and 35 percent wheat protein concentrate (enzyme inactivated).
[b] Mineral premix contains tricalcium phosphate, ferrous fumarate, zinc sulfate and iodized salt.
[c] Vitamin premix contains vitamin A palmitate (stabilized), vitamin D (stabilized), alpha-tocopherol acetate, thiamine mononitrate, ascorbic acid (ethyl cellulose-coated), pyridoxine hydrochloride, niacin, calcium D-pantothenate, folic acid, and vitamin B12 in a soy flour carrier.

SOURCE: USDA/CCC Announcements WSB11 and CSB8, February 20, 1996.

TABLE 1-2. Selected Nutrient Composition of Corn–Soy Blend (CSB)

	Nutrients in CSB Components				
Nutrient	Corn Meal (gelatinized degermed) (69.8 g)	Soy Flour (defatted) (21.9 g)	Soy Oil (5.5 g)	Vit/Min[a] Premix (2.8 g)	Total Nutrient Per 100g CSB
Energy (Kcal)	259	72.0	48.6	—	379.6
Protein (g)	5.92	11.24	—	—	17.16
Calcium (mg)	3.5	52.7	—	744	800
Phosphorus (mg)	38.7	147.3	—	400	586
Iron (mg)	0.77	2.02	—	15.2	17.99
Sodium (mg)	13.96	4.38	—	254.0	272.3
Zinc (mg)	0.5	0.54	—	0.9	1.94
Iodine (mg)	—	—	—	45.5	45.5
Vitamin A (IU)	288	0.80	—	2,314	2,603
Vitamin D (IU)	—	—	—	198	198
Vitamin E (mg)	0.23	0.042	—	7.5	7.8
Vitamin C (mg)	—	—	—	40	40
Thiamine (mg)	0.098	0.153	—	0.28	0.53
Riboflavin (mg)	0.035	0.055	—	0.39	0.48
Niacin (mg)	0.70	0.571	—	4.9	6.17
Pantothenic acid (mg)	0.218	0.436	—	2.75	3.42
Pyridoxine (mg)	0.18	0.125	—	0.165	0.47
Folacin (mcg)	33.5	66.7	—	198	298
Vitamin B12 (mcg)	—	—	—	3.97	3.97

[a] Vitamin and mineral premix USDA/CCC 1996 specifications.

SOURCE: Calculations based on USDA, Agricultural Research Service. 1997. USDA Nutrient Database for Standard Reference, Release 11-1 (**http://www.nal.usda.gov/fnic/foodcomp**)

TABLE 1-3. Selected Nutrient Composition of Wheat–Soy Blend (WSB)

	Nutrients in WSB Components				
Nutrient	Wheat Fractions[a] (73.1 g)	Soy Flour Defatted (20 g)	Soy Oil (5.5 g)	Vit/min[b] Premix 2.9 g	Total Nutrient per 100 g WSB
Energy (kcal)	250	65.8	48.62	—	364.4
Protein (g)	10.0	9.4	—	—	19.4
Calcium (mg)	25.6	48.2	—	744	818
Phosphorus (mg)	219.3	134.7	—	400	754
Iron (mg)	1.8	1.8	—	15.2	18.8
Sodium (mg)	211	4	—	254	469
Zinc (mg)	1.41	0.49	—	0.9	2.8
Iodine (mg)	—	—	—	45.5	45.5
Vitamin A (IU)	—	8	—	2,314	2,322
Vitamin D (IU)	—	—	—	198	198
Vitamin E (mg)	0.12	0.4	1.0	7.5	9.02
Vitamin C (mg)	—	—	—	40	40
Thiamine (mg)	0.17	0.14	—	0.28	0.59
Riboflavin (mg)	0.08	0.05	—	0.39	0.52
Niacin (mg)	3.74	0.52	—	4.9	9.16
Patothenic acid (mg)	0.76	0.40	—	2.75	3.91
Pyridoxine (mg)	0.25	0.11	—	0.165	0.525
Folacin (mcg)	19.7	61.1	—	198	278.8
Vitamin B_{12} (mcg)	—	—	—	3.97	3.97

[a] Wheat fractions nutrient content based on bulgur only.
[b] Vitamin and mineral premix USDA/CCC 1996 specifications.

SOURCE: Calculations based on USDA, Agricultural Research Service. 1997. USDA Nutrient Database for Standard Reference, Release 11-1 (**http://www.nal.usda.gov/fnic/foodcomp**).

These highly fortified blended foods are provided as ration supplements to refugees and displaced persons in camps and to beneficiaries of developmental aid programs that are targeted largely to mothers and children. (Developmental aid uses food primarily in school feeding programs, in maternal and child health programs, and in food-for-work projects where the food is used as a substitute for money to pay for labor on development projects. Developmental food aid is rarely the sole source of food for the family.) These blended, cereal-based foods are partially precooked during processing, which allows them to be incorporated easily into a number of different food preparations that are acceptable to many different cultures and to be prepared by the recipient with a minimal use of fuel.

It has been estimated that 44 percent of global food aid deliveries were financed by the United States in 1996. However, the United States supplied 84 percent of the total blended, fortified foods used worldwide (Dr. Judit Katone-Apte, World Food Programme, United Nations, personal communication, 1997). Of the blended, fortified food commodities provided by the United States in majority of this (75 percent) going to India for development feeding programs. Only 18 percent of U.S.-supplied CSB and WSB went to Africa (USAID, 1997 a, b).

Beginning in fiscal year (FY) 1993, U.S. congressional appropriations committees urged USAID to increase the amount of vitamin C (L-ascorbic acid) added to blended commodities exported through the P.L. 480 Title II Food for Peace program to levels more than twice those currently in use (Foreign Operations, Export Financing, and Related Programs Appropriations Bill, 1993, S. Rpt. 102-419, 1994, S. Rpt. 103-142) (see Appendix A). The commodities targeted for increased fortification with vitamin C were CSB and WSB—the only commodities exported in the Food for Peace program that are fortified with vitamin C. The stated purpose of the increased vitamin C fortification of these blended foods was to improve the health of food aid recipients and reduce the need for, and cost of, later medical interventions (Foreign Operations, Export Financing, and Related Programs Appropriations Bill, 1994, S. Rpt. 103-142). The 1995 congressional report asked for information on the cost of the increased fortification and the stability of vitamin C throughout the shipping process (Making Appropriations for the Foreign Operations, Export Financing, and Related Programs for the fiscal year ending September 30, 1995, Conference Report, H. Rpt. 103-633, 1995).

In response to the original 1993 congressional appropriations bill language, USAID's Bureau for Humanitarian Response (BHR) commissioned an examination of the various options for appropriate micronutrient fortification of USAID food aid commodities. The resulting technical review paper *Micronutrient Fortification and Enrichment of P.L. 480 Title II Commodities: Recommendations for Improvement* (OMNI, 1994) addressed fortification with many nutrients, including vitamin C, and provided cost information. That report, as well as Toole (1994), documented that the most widespread micronutrient deficiencies are iron deficiency anemia, which occurs worldwide, and vitamin A deficiency, which is endemic in South Asia and in eastern and southern Africa. Iodine deficiency also exists in most regions of the world, whereas deficiencies of vitamin C, niacin, and thiamin tend to be infrequent and very localized. The 1994 OMNI (Opportunities for Micronutrient Intervention) report recommended that vitamin C fortification levels be maintained at 40 mg/100 g until further information became available on the stability of vitamin C during storage and preparation. In response, Hoffmann La-Roche, Inc. (a vitamin manufacturer), submitted comments on the recommendations, including the following, "Of particular concern is the inconsistency of supplementation levels and the inadequacy of the vitamin C supplementation in exported grains."[1] USAID was

---

[1] Rita Norton, Vice President for Federal Government Affairs, Hoffmann-LaRoche, Inc. to Robert Kramer, Food for Peace Program, May 11, 1995.

able to obtain some analyses of the vitamin C content of blended foods,[2] but information was lacking on how much vitamin C actually reaches the recipient at the time of food preparation and consumption.

The stability of vitamin C (L-ascorbic acid) is of concern because this is one of the most labile vitamins in foods. Its main loss during processing and storage is from oxidation, which is accelerated by light, oxygen, heat, increased pH, high moisture content (water activity), and the presence of copper or ferrous salts. To reduce oxidation, the vitamin C used in commodity fortification is coated with ethyl cellulose (2.5 percent). Oxidative losses also occur during food processing and preparation, and additional vitamin C may be lost if it dissolves into cooking liquid and is then discarded.

The FY 1996 Senate Appropriations Committee Report 104-143, "Foreign Operations, Export Financing, and Related Programs Appropriation Bill, 1996," directed USAID to initiate a pilot program to increase the vitamin C content of CSB and WSB to 90 mg per 100 g and to report on the results (Appendix A). In response, USAID set up a cooperative agreement with the organization SUSTAIN (Sharing United States Technology to Aid in the Improvement of Nutrition) to devise and implement the pilot program. USAID also asked the Institute of Medicine to form a committee to address the cost-effectiveness and advisability of increasing the level of vitamin C used to fortify the food aid commodities CSB and WSB. The Committee on International Nutrition— Vitamin C in Food Aid Commodities was constituted in response to this request.

THE COMMITTEE'S TASK

The committee's overall task was to address the cost-effectiveness and advisability of scaling up vitamin C fortification of the Title II commodities CSB and WSB to improve recipients' diet, nutrition, and health. First, the committee was to review the proposed pilot program, examining it for soundness of scientific and technical design in relation to (1) monitoring the presence and stability of vitamin C in food aid commodities and (2) assessing the dietary intake of vitamin C, nutritional status, and health status of recipients. Based on this review, the committee was to prepare a brief report to recommend modifications needed to improve the pilot program's design.

For this final report, the committee's specific role was to assess the results of the pilot program; estimate the need for increased vitamin C fortification to improve recipient diet, nutrition, and health; and estimate the cost-effectiveness of increased fortification with vitamin C. In addition, this report provides recommendations regarding both the advisability of scaling up Title II

---

[2] Robert K. Boyer, Food for Peace Program, to the Honorable H.L. Livingston, Narrative on Conference Report, March 1, 1995.

commodity fortification with vitamin C and the appropriateness of this approach compared with other means of delivering vitamin C.

THE STUDY PROCESS

The committee met twice during the study. Prior to and during the first meeting, committee members reviewed *The Vitamin C Pilot Program* (Ranum and Chomé, 1996), excerpts from the report *Micronutrient Fortification and Enrichment of P.L. 480 Title II Commodities: Recommendations for Improvement, Technical Review Paper* (OMNI, 1994), and a variety of other materials. An open session with representatives of USAID and SUSTAIN, USDA, the Food and Drug Administration, Kellogg Corporation, and Protein Grain Products International was also held. The committee then deliberated in executive session and prepared its report *Vitamin C in Food Aid Commodities: Initial Review of a Pilot Program* (IOM, 1996). In particular, the report reviewed the plan for the pilot program designed by SUSTAIN, presented recommendations for its improvement, and identified additional information needed to complete the overall task. The committee emphasized the potential value of collecting data from emergency feeding programs, as well as from development programs, and of collecting samples on-site to determine vitamin C losses during food preparation. It also stressed the need for cost data and information on both the prevalence of scurvy and insufficient vitamin C and iron intakes in populations that receive blended foods. SUSTAIN had access to the committee's initial report as it completed its pilot program.

The committee staff, under committee guidance, conducted an extensive literature search to attain a more global view of the reported incidence of scurvy in refugee populations, the effects of vitamin C on iron absorption, and other potential health effects of increased vitamin C supplementation. The committee also contacted the United Nations World Food Programme (WFP) for additional information on the vitamin C status of food aid recipients.

Prior to and during its second meeting, the committee reviewed SUSTAIN's report *Results Report on the Vitamin C Pilot Program* (Ranum and Chomé, 1997) and assessed needs for additional information. An open session was held by videoconference with representatives of USAID and SUSTAIN. Information on the tonnage of CSB and WSB produced and their distribution in development versus emergency relief programs was obtained, along with information on costs of the various methods of providing vitamin C. The committee teleconferenced with a UN representative for additional insights into global food aid needs.

This range of activities provided the committee with the information on which it based its deliberations. This report presents the results of the committee's analyses and deliberations, as well as its conclusions and recommendations. This chapter provides the background for the study and the committee's charge. Chapter 2 focuses on the prevalence of scurvy, vitamin C requirements, and the role of vitamin C in other aspects of human health. Chapter 3 presents cost-effectiveness analysis of vitamin C fortification. Chapter 4 summarizes pilot program results, and Chapter 5 contains the committee's critique of the pilot program. The committee's conclusions and recommendations are presented in Chapter 6.

2

Vitamin C: Needs and Functions

Vitamin C (L-ascorbic acid and its reduced form, dehydroascorbic acid) is a water-soluble vitamin whose best-defined function is as a cofactor for the enzyme required in the hydroxylation of proline and lysine in collagen formation. It can be synthesized by many mammals, but not by humans. The highest vitamin C content is found in green and red peppers, broccoli, citrus fruits, strawberries, melons, tomatoes, raw cabbage, potatoes, and leafy greens such as spinach, turnip, and mustard greens. Meat, fish, poultry, eggs, and dairy products contain much smaller amounts, and cereal grains contain essentially none. Losses of vitamin C occur when foods are cooked in large amounts of water, exposed to extensive heating, or exposed to air.

Dietary deficiency of vitamin C eventually leads to scurvy, a serious disease characterized by the weakening of collagenous structures that results in widespread capillary hemorrhaging (Hornig, 1975; Woodruff, 1975). Clinical signs of scurvy, including swollen or bleeding gums, petechial hemorrhages, joint pain, and follicular hyperkeratosis, are associated with plasma (or serum) vitamin C values of less than 0.2 mg/dl (Hodges et al., 1969, 1971). Minimum dietary vitamin C intakes ranging from 6.5 to 10 mg per day were required to cure clinical signs of scurvy. When levels ranging from 6.5 to 130.5 mg daily were administered to adult males showing multiple clinical signs of scurvy, the rate of recovery from its signs and symptoms was proportional to the dose of vitamin C (Baker et al., 1971). Higher doses (32 to 600 mg/day) were needed for the most rapid improvement of symptoms in adult males (Hodges et al., 1969; Baker et al., 1971).

PREVALENCE OF SCURVY

The United Nations Subcommittee on Nutrition reported that nearly 200 million children under 5 years of age continue to be malnourished. In some regions, such as sub-Saharan Africa and South Asia, the lack of nutritional improvement combined with the rapid rise in population has resulted in an actual increase in the total number of malnourished children. Most of sub-Saharan Africa is now worse off nutritionally than 10 years ago. At the same time, global food aid deliveries have been continuously reduced since 1993 (ACC/SCN, 1997).

There are no data available on the prevalence of scurvy in free-living populations worldwide. The Centers for Disease Control and Prevention (CDC, 1992) indicated that scurvy has been rarely reported in stable populations in developing countries. Global dietary intake data to assess the prevalence of low vitamin C intakes are also lacking. However, Seaman and Rivers (1989) noted that in Central and South America and in Southeast Asia, refugees generally either receive diets adequate in vitamin C or are able to obtain them via trade, cultivation, or other income.

There is evidence of the outbreak of scurvy among refugee populations entirely dependent on emergency relief rations that provide less than 2 mg of vitamin C per day per person. Scurvy outbreaks have been reported in refugee populations during the past three decades, mainly in East Africa (CDC, 1989, 1992; Desenclos et al., 1989; ACC/SCN, 1996). The greatest number of outbreaks occurred in the 1980s in Somalia. Notably, no outbreaks have been reported from West and Central African refugee populations located in Liberia, Sierra Leone, the Great Lakes of Central Africa, and Angola.

Actual numbers of scurvy cases are difficult to assess, mainly because of the lack of adequate surveillance systems in refugee camps. Mortality rates may also be high among vitamin C-deficient individuals, who are likely to suffer from other severe vitamin and mineral deficiencies and to be at increased risk of morbidity and mortality from infectious diseases. Thus, the estimates of 100,000 cases of scurvy among refugee populations in East Africa (Somalia, Sudan, Ethiopia and Kenya) in the late 1970s through the 1980s may have been an under-estimate, to some extent, of the magnitude of the problem at that time (Desenclos et al., 1989).

Four outbreaks of scruvy have been reported since 1994, when the World Food Programme (WFP) and the United Nations High Commissioner for Refugees (UNHCR) adopted the policy of providing fortified, blended foods to populations wholly dependent on food aid, in an effort to preempt any micronutrient deficiencies. One outbreak occurred in Rwandan refugees in eastern Zaire in the spring of 1994 prior to the time that the newly adopted food aid plan could be implemented. Recurring mild incidences of scurvy were reported among Bhutanese refugees in Nepal in 1994, 1995, and 1996, and moderate outbreaks were reported among Somalian refugees in the Dadaab camp in Kenya in 1994 and 1996. However, since the initial cases appeared in June and peaked around September, the scurvy outbreaks in the Dadaab camp appeared to be seasonal rather than related to the distribution of fortified, blended foods. This corresponded to a lack of fresh food and high prices for camel's milk. Purchased camel's milk, wild foods, and fruits and vegetables from kitchen gardens are generally the main sources of vitamin C for this population. Withdrawal of the fortified, blended food from the general ration when supplies ran out did not change the pattern of scurvy occurrence in 1996 (Van Nieuwenhuyse, 1997, as reported by Ranum and Chomé, 1997). It is not clear whether those with scurvy had received any of the fortified, blended food and, if they did, that the amount received was sufficient so that doubling the vitamin C fortification would have made a difference. Thus, the potential protective effect of fortified blends is difficult to assess. In addition, the scurvy outbreak among Somali refugees in Kenya in 1994 was reported even though they received 50 g per day of CSB which is expected to provide 20 mg of vitamin C (Van Nieuwennhuyse, 1997, as reported by Ranum and Chomé, 1997). It was believed that no vitamin C remained after preparation because the recipients cooked the CSB more than 30 minutes. Further, data from the pilot program indicate the strong possibility that the CSB did not contain the specified levels of vitamin C.

In most scurvy outbreak situations, the main contributing factor has been a dependence on standard emergency relief rations, which until 1994 consisted of a cereal flour, vegetable oil, pulses, and occasionally salt, and contained almost no vitamin C (< 2 mg per person per day), and the limited availability of local supplies of fresh produce (Toole, 1994). Transportation and accessibility problems, inefficient markets, drought, seasonal shortages, and the inability to cultivate or to trade for other food sources have been identified as the main factors contributing to scurvy outbreaks. In such situations, outbreaks of scurvy have occurred within 3 to 4 months of exclusive consumption of emergency relief rations (Magan et al., 1983; Desenclos et al., 1989). In refugee camps, the risk of developing scurvy increased with length of residence and age and was greater among females, particularly pregnant and lactating women (Desenclos et al., 1989).

Until 1994, fortified cereal blends were provided only occasionally in general relief rations because these blends were normally reserved for targeted supplemental feeding programs (Toole, 1994). They were about twice as expensive as the plain milled cereals normally distributed in general rations (UNHCR, 1989). Only in 1994 was a policy adopted by the WFP and the UNHCR to distribute fortified cereals in the early stage of an emergency situation or to populations totally dependent on food aid.

VITAMIN C REQUIREMENTS

In food fortification, the amounts of nutrients added should be sufficient to maintain nutritional status. Considerably higher quantities of nutrients will be needed to cure existing deficiencies and replete nutrient stores. The level of ascorbic acid in blended, fortified commodities (40 mg/100 g) was based on the 1974 National Research Council (NRC) recommendations for children up to 11 years of age, by assuming an intake of 100 g of blended cereal per day (Dr. Samuel Kahn, USAID, personal communication, September, 1997). Current rations of blended, fortified commodities vary with the specific situation but in emergency feeding situations are usually 30 g per person per day. The blended, fortified commodities are not intended to be the sole or even major source of nutrients because 30 g per day will provide only 114 kcal, or 5–6 percent of daily energy requirements, and 5–6 g of protein.

The current Recommended Dietary Allowances (RDAs) in the United States for vitamin C are: 40 mg at 1–3 years of age, 45 mg at 3–6 years of age, 60 mg for adult men and women, 70 mg for pregnancy, and 90–95 mg during lactation (NRC, 1989). The Food and Agriculture Organization (FAO)/World Health Organization (WHO, 1993) has estimated that the average requirements for vitamin C are 20–25 mg per day from age 2.5 through adult years, 35 mg per day in pregnancy, and 55 mg per day during lactation. Substantially less than the recommended intake is needed to prevent scurvy in adults. From 6.5 to 10 mg of vitamin C per day is the most frequently cited amount necessary to prevent overt scurvy. Body pools are depleted rapidly (3 percent per day) when vitamin C intake is low (Baker et al., 1971; Irwin and Hutchins, 1976; NRC, 1989). Outbreaks of scurvy were reported in Ethiopia when intake averaged 2 mg per day (Toole, 1992).

It has been estimated that 29 mg of vitamin C per 1000 kilocalories (kcal) is an adequate minimal concentration that will cover the requirements of all groups and promote iron absorption (Beaton, 1995). This value is based on the level of vitamin C necessary to maintain stores during periods of inadequate intake. School children in Egypt and Kenya consumed 34 and 39 mg/1000 kcal respectively, whereas in Mexico, children's intakes were lower, 12 mg/1000 kcal and none were scorbutic (Calloway et al., 1993). The average intake of 2 mg per day that resulted in scurvy outbreaks in Ethiopia corresponded to approximately 1–3 mg/1000 kcal.

Based on the FAO/WHO recommended intake of 30 mg of ascorbic acid per day and the assumption that 40 g of CSB is consumed by children (OMNI, 1994), CSB fortified at the current level could provide about half of the recommended amount of vitamin C (16 mg per day). Although this is significantly higher than the intakes associated with scurvy outbreaks, it does not account for cooking losses.

OTHER FUNCTIONS OF VITAMIN C

Vitamin C has other functions in addition to its role in collagen synthesis. Along with its role in hydroxylation reactions, vitamin C affects leukocyte (Anderson and Theron, 1979) and macrophage (Anderson and Lukey, 1987) function, immune response (Leibovitz and Siegel, 1978), wound healing (Levenson et al., 1971), and allergic reactions (Dawson and West, 1965). The involvement of vitamin C in these areas is less well documented, and the levels necessary to achieve these benefits are not known but are assumed to be much higher (pharmacological) than those required for scurvy prevention. Thus, the priority for adding vitamin C based on these roles cannot be established. However, if cost-effectiveness analyses show that providing higher fortification levels to prevent scurvy is not warranted, it is extremely unlikely that better knowledge about the other possible benefits of vitamin C would result in favorable cost-effective analysis for this objective.

VITAMIN C AND IRON ABSORPTION

Vitamin C in the diet can enhance the absorption of iron from plant sources (non-heme iron) and improve the absorbability of fortification iron (nonchelated inorganic iron) added to diets that contain inhibitors of iron absorption (e.g., the phytate and polyphenols found in CSB and WSB). The effects of ascorbic acid and of foods containing the same amount of ascorbic acid appear to be the same. A two to threefold increase in absorption of non-heme food iron from a meal can be expected from adding foods that contain about 50–100 mg of ascorbic acid (Hallberg et al., 1987). In the past few years, concern about the prevalence of iron deficiency anemia in recipient populations (which is undoubtedly vastly higher than the prevalence of ascorbic acid deficiency) has provoked recommendations to increase the present level of iron in commodities from 15 to 30 mg/kg (OMNI, 1994). However, this may result in organoleptic problems, as well as accelerated ascorbic acid oxidation during storage. It is the committee's understanding that the feasibility of increasing the ferrous fumarate content of WSB and CSB is as yet unresolved. However, the efficiency of absorption of ferrous iron added to CSB is likely to be relatively poor (Cook et al., 1984). The addition of about 25 mg of ascorbic acid to a meal approximately doubles the percentage of non-heme iron absorbed (Cook and Monson, 1977; Allen and Ahluwalia, 1997). However, data on the effect of increased levels of vitamin C added to corn–soy milk (CSM) showed no significant improvement in iron absorption (Dr. Sean Lynch, personal communication, September 1997).

An alternate recommendation was made in *Technical Review of Vitamin C and Iron Levels in PL 480 II Commodities* (USAID, 1990). The action recommended was to change the fortificant from ferrous fumarate to an iron-EDTA (ethylenediaminetetraacetic acid) chelate based on the fact that this would improve iron absorption substantially, and eliminate the need for high vitamin C levels to facilitate iron absorption. (In the same review, an increase in vitamin C content was not recommended because the moisture content of commodities had been shown to promote destruction of vitamin C. It was recommended that the manufacturers' capability to lower the moisture content of the commodities be examined.) Unlike ferrous fumarate, an iron-EDTA chelate would not contribute to the oxidation of ascorbic acid during storage.

3

Cost-Effectiveness Analysis

The assessment of cost-effectiveness depends on measuring the effectiveness along with the cost of an intervention. The most useful application of cost-effectiveness analysis is to compare alternative interventions in terms of a given level of a particular effect. One of the complicating factors in cost-effectiveness analysis is that an intervention (e.g., raising the level of vitamin C fortification) may have several effects; it may be highly cost-effective for some of these effects but not others. Cost-effectiveness analysis cannot help assess which effect should be given priority.

EFFECTIVENESS

Measures of effectiveness depend on the objectives of a project. The current pilot project implicitly identifies two objectives: (1) to improve or maintain the vitamin C status of the target (beneficiary) population and (2) improve or maintain the iron status of the population by providing vitamin C to enhance iron absorption. It is assumed that accomplishing these will achieve the congressionally mandated objective of improving the health of food aid recipients, thereby reducing the need for, and cost of, later medical interventions. The first objective, improving or maintaining the vitamin C intake of the target population, seems to consist of two subobjectives: (1) to cure scurvy in populations where the deficiency disease is present and (2) to prevent its occurrence by ensuring the dietary sufficiency of vitamin C.

A secondary objective is to improve the iron status of the target population. The implicit assumption is that adding additional vitamin C to corn–soy blend (CSB) or wheat–soy blend (WSB) is an appropriate way to achieve this objective. Cost-effectiveness assessment ideally would compare the chosen pilot

23

intervention with alternatives (e.g., raising the *iron* fortification level; changing the type of iron used). However, reviewing iron fortification levels was not part of this committee's task.

Both objectives of the pilot study involve improving the micronutrient status of a target population. The benefit to be gained from the project depends on raising the population from a state of vitamin C deficiency to a state of vitamin C sufficiency. *There is no benefit to be gained from raising the population's intake or absorption of a nutrient if the amount is already satisfactory.* Thus, the measures of effectiveness depend not only on the success of nutrient delivery to, and consumption by, a target population but also on the previous status of the population.

U.S. food aid is used for two purposes: developmental aid and emergency relief. Approximately 88 percent of U.S.-supplied fortified, blended food is used for developmental purposes. Developmental aid uses food primarily in school feeding programs, maternal and child health (MCH) programs, and food-for-work projects where the food is used as a substitute for money to pay for labor on development projects. Developmental food aid is rarely the sole source of food for a family, and since there is no evidence of vitamin C deficiency in populations receiving this type of food aid there is no rationale for increasing vitamin C in food aid commodities for this purpose.

Many recipients of developmental food aid are iron deficient (OMNI, 1994; Toole, 1994; Beaton, 1995). However, doubling the vitamin C content of fortified, blended foods to improve iron absorption may be much less cost-effective than increasing the iron content of such foods above their present levels of fortification, or of increasing iron in the diet by other means. Research data to support either intervention are insufficient.

Emergency relief food aid is distributed to refugees and other distressed populations (famine sufferers or other displaced populations) in camps. A small proportion of refugee populations has been shown to be vitamin C deficient when unfortified food was given (Ranum and Chomé, 1997). All of these populations were in the eastern Sahel (greater Horn of Africa and Kenya)., Except for some recent reports of Bhutanese refugees in Nepal, no other refugee populations have shown documented evidence of vitamin C deficiency, including many others in the rest of Africa.

If the proposal under consideration is to increase the fortification levels of vitamin C in all CSB and WSB, then the cost of such an intervention must be measured against the small number of beneficiaries who are actually in need of the nutrient. For any project of a given size and cost, the cost-effectiveness is lower (that is, better) if the proportion of the population in need is higher.

The cost-effectiveness analysis uses as a basis for comparison the nutrient content of blended foods at present levels of fortification that could *not* be purchased under the Public Law (P.L.) 480 Title II program because the money was spent increasing the vitamin C fortification. This is a conservative basis for comparison because the nutrient content of other usual food aid commodities that could not be bought would be many times greater, resulting in analyses that are much less favorable to increased fortification. Although this analysis is based on the assumption of a fixed dollar amount available for purchase of blended foods, the results are not dependent on this assumption because the same principles apply to any increases in funding that might be allocated specifically to increased vitamin C fortification instead of increased food aid.

Although outbreaks of scurvy in refugee populations are a concern, both inadequate food intake (in part alleviated by the blended commodities) and a high prevalence of other micronutrient deficiencies are also common problems. For example, deficiencies of niacin, iron, vitamin A, and iodine also occur in these populations (OMNI, 1994; Toole, 1994). Thus, the benefits of increased expenditures on vitamin C have to be viewed in the context of asking why adding more of this nutrient is more important than supplementing with other nutrients or simply increasing the total amount of blended, fortified food provided.

Vitamin C Objective

Scurvy has not been documented among stable, free-living populations that are the typical target group for development projects, except in extreme situations of famine. Scurvy has been documented in a small proportion of refugee camps in the greater Horn of Africa. It was found only under the most adverse conditions: isolated camps entirely dependent on food aid rations, with no possibility of trade or exchange with local markets and with no time to grow their own foods or adapt to the local situation. Three outbreaks have occurred in this high risk area (Kenya, Ethiopia, Sudan) since the World Food Programme (WFP) and the United Nations High Commissioner for Refugees (UNHCR) adopted the policy in 1994 of providing fortified, blended foods to populations wholly dependent on food aid. Other risk factors for scurvy include physiological status (pregnancy and lactation), and, in some cases, length of time traveling to a camp and conditions during transit. This describes only a small proportion of all the refugees in camps in which rations are provided; many have access to local indigenous markets, and some camps have provision for refugees growing small amounts of food themselves.

Food rations delivered in development programs (e.g., MCH supplementary feeding, school feeding, etc.) are intended as supplements, not as complete diets. In these free-living populations, access to markets and/or home-produced food is a given assumption. Vitamin C deficiency has rarely been reported in such populations.

Iron Objective

The same considerations apply to iron. Iron deficiency has been far more widely documented as a nutritional problem than scurvy, both in the artificial environment of refugee camps and in the low-income, free-living populations that would be the beneficiaries of developmental food aid. In terms of this objective, the question for cost-effectiveness analysis is whether adding vitamin C to the diet through CSB and WSB is the most cost effective way to achieve improved iron status.

COST

Cost-effectiveness analysis typically considers *all* the costs involved in a given intervention, including (for food distribution) raw materials, processing, transport, and the labor of people involved in the distribution and preparation of the food. For example, if a food required additional preparation time, the cost of that time (although not an accounting cost to the project) would be included. If all CSB and WSB were fortified with vitamin C at the higher level, the food would be handled, transported, stored, distributed, and prepared in exactly the same way as before; only the additional cost of vitamin C in the premix would be considered a program cost. There are no side effects from high doses of vitamin C even at the maximum intakes possible if fortification levels are doubled. Thus the cost of potential side effects does not have to be taken into account.

According to the Sharing United States Technology to Aid in the Improvement of Nutrition (SUSTAIN) report (Ranum and Chomé, 1997), the U.S. Agency for International Development (USAID) considers it operationally very difficult for the U.S. P.L. 480 program to add extra vitamin C to only some of the CSB or WSB in the program and then to target the blends containing extra fortification toward emergency populations identified as likely to benefit. There is also a considerable lag time involved in procuring and shipping such special foods, typically 4 to 6 months (see Boxes 4-1, 4-2). If this lag time cannot be reduced, the provision of specially prepared, high vitamin C blended foods is an inappropriate response to emergency needs for additional vitamin C, although it may be appropriate when the risk of low vitamin C intake continues.

The cost-effectiveness assessment would be affected if it were possible to fortify a small percentage of blended food and target this food specifically to refugee situations known to be at high risk of vitamin C deficiency over the long run. Cost-effectiveness would be improved because the additional fortification would be required only for the small percentage of blended food going to the high-risk population; however, there would be some additional management cost involved in keeping track of two separate supplies of blended food. Those responsible for such commodities at USAID's Bureau of Humanitarian Response (BHR) suggested that this would be quite difficult to do.

COST-EFFECTIVENESS ESTIMATE

Vitamin C Objective

The objective of raising blended foods' fortification levels is to avert vitamin C deficiency or scurvy. Thus, the proper measure of cost-effectiveness is the *cost per case of scurvy averted.* For food relief programs, the recommended daily allowance of vitamin C is 30 mg (FAO/WHO, 1974) but the majority of references cited in this report (Barker et al., 1971; Hodges et al., 1969, 1971) state that an intake of 6–10 mg per day is sufficient to prevent the appearance of symptoms of vitamin C deficiency in a population.

The cost per case of scurvy averted could not be measured directly. There have been no representative studies of scurvy incidence or prevalence in refugee populations, only anecdotal reports and localized (single camp) surveys of scurvy outbreaks in particular locations. The following analysis is based on the assumptions spelled out in the text and is in this sense a hypothetical "best guess." The conclusion is that using the most optimistic assumptions, the cost of using highly fortified CSB to avert a case of scurvy may range from $158 to $1,223, depending entirely on assumptions regarding coverage of the target population, while the cost to avert a case of scurvy by tripling the conventional ration may range from $7.45 to $74.50 based on the expectation that rations would be targeted by camp, but not by individual within a camp. Thus increasing the conventional ration to high-risk camps is at least 2.1 times more cost-effective than increasing the level of fortification and may be 16.4 times as cost-effective or more.

Assumptions Regarding Proportion of Beneficiaries at Risk of Vitamin C Deficiency and Scurvy: Size of the Target Population

The objective of the project is not to deliver vitamin C; it is to avert vitamin C deficiency, specifically scurvy. Delivery of vitamin C to populations already sufficient in vitamin C is a waste. Although the possibility always exists that there may be unknown benefits to consuming levels of nutrients above those known to be needed for good health, it is not reasonable to make a program priority of this uncertain benefit when so many other known needs are present. According to data provided in the SUSTAIN report and elsewhere (Toole, 1994), scurvy is rarely seen in stable, free-living populations. Vitamin C is not among the high-priority micronutrients identified as a public health concern in less developed countries (OMNI, 1994). Even in emergency feeding situations, documented scurvy outbreaks are uncommon in refugee camps in Latin America and Asia; in Africa, the majority of reported outbreaks of scurvy have been in the Eastern Sahel (greater Horn of Africa and Kenya).

Seventy-five percent of blended foods provided by the United States go to India (USAID, 1997a, b). All of this is used in development programs targeted primarily towards maternal and child health supplementary feeding. An additional 7 percent goes to development programs in Central and South America. Of the remaining 18 percent, much is distributed in development programs. On the assumption that half of this 18 percent goes to refugee feeding at most, it can be estimated that 9–10 percent of blended foods are distributed in refugee and emergency feeding programs. Not more than 70 percent of these applications are likely to be in East Africa, where scurvy has been reported. This means that only 7 percent of blended foods at most are distributed in situations where vitamin C deficiency might be a problem.

TABLE 3-1 Possible Consequences of Added Cost from Higher Vitamin C Levels

	CSB	WSB	Total
Quantity purchased (MT)	238,300	11,310	249,610
Total cost ($)	79,768,542	5,184,617	84,953,159
Average cost ($/MT)	334.74	458.41	—
Average cost ($/bag)	18.41	25.21	—
Extra vitamin Cost ($/MT)	6.33	6.33	—
Total extra cost ($)	1,508,439	71,592	1,580,031
Equivalent product (MT)[a]	4,506	156	—
Fewer people/year at 30g/person/day	411,534	14,263	425,797
Cost of product reaching at risk individuals ($/MT)[b]	Range: $90 to $3,610		

[a] The amount of product that could not be distributed if the cost of the increase in vitamin C (from 40 to 90 mg) was subtracted from the total amount of funds available during FY 1996 to produce these commodities.

[b] Based on assumptions that only 7 percent of blended foods reach refugee camps in East Africa, and the percentage of individuals in these camps who are at risk of deficiency was 25 percent and 10 percent.

SOURCE: Adapted from Ranum and Chomé, 1997.

Thus, fully 93 percent of the cost of adding more vitamin C to blended food as a strategy for avoiding scurvy would likely be unnecessary in nutritional terms. In monetary terms, the marginal cost to provide additional fortification of blended foods is $6.33/MT (Table 3-1). The marginal cost of fortifying blended foods likely to reach refugee populations in East Africa is $90.43/MT (27 percent of the current price). Since not all of this group is at risk, the cost per actual target beneficiary reached could be much higher. For example, if 25 percent of East African refugee camps are at high risk of deficiency, the marginal cost of reaching a target camp by fortifying all blended food with high levels of vitamin C is $361 per MT that actually reaches the target population. These high costs result from the inability to target fortified food to the at-risk population. If 10 percent of the at-risk population is actually deficient in vitamin C, the cost of reaching the deficient group is ten times this, or $3,610/MT. That is, based on these assumptions, to deliver one dollar's worth of vitamin C through fortified food to the target individual would require distribution of $40 worth of food: only one fourth ($10) reaches the high-risk camps, and of this only one tenth ($1) actually reaches the deficient individual. Alternative strategies that can target individuals with deficient vitamin C intake could be much more cost-effective, even if the cost per target individual were higher because the leakage to individuals not in need of the intervention would be lower.

Our interest, however, is not so much in the cost per MT of food delivered to the target population, but in the cost per case of scurvy averted. To estimate this requires an estimate of the total size of the population at risk. Although the incidence of scurvy can be high in isolated instances, the total number of reported cases over the past 20 years is about 100,000 (Desenclos et al., 1989), or only 5,000 cases per year. It is likely that the incidence of scurvy is underreported, but doubling the incidence yields an estimate of only 10,000 cases per year, representing a very small proportion (0.06%) of the estimated 17 million refugees per year depending on food aid (Toole, 1992). At current levels of P.L. 480 distribution, the quantity of blended food going to refugees in camps is enough to provide a 30 g daily ration to 13% of the total number of refugees in camps, or 2.21 million people per year. This number represents more than 200 times the estimated scurvy incidence of 10,000 cases, although there is no assurance that normal distribution would necessarily target those individuals.

Assumptions Regarding Nutrient Losses

The SUSTAIN pilot study estimated losses of vitamin C from conventional and highly fortified blends. It showed losses of zero to 13 percent during transport and storage, which can be considered negligible. However, losses in cooking are much more significant.

At high levels of fortification, retention of vitamin C after cooking CSB was between 48 percent and 67 percent (see Table 4-2). The higher figure was for blends fortified to a level of 170 mg/100 g, much higher than the highest level of fortification proposed, therefore that figure was not used in subsequent calculations. The lower figure was fairly consistent for blends fortified at around 100 mg/100 g, which is close to the proposed level of 90 mg/100 g. Therefore, the lower figure (48 percent) is used in these estimates. Retention of vitamin C in highly fortified WSB was lower, 32–33 percent (see Table 4-3). At conventional levels of fortification, CSB was estimated to retain 17 to 32 percent (average 24.5 percent) of vitamin C. Although these results are questionable, they are the best available empirical estimates. Conventionally fortified WSB retained about 18 percent of its vitamin C content. For purposes of these estimates, the figures for CSB are used, which represents more than 95 percent of the total blended food provided under P.L. 480.

With these estimated retentions (24.5 and 48 percent), 100 g of CSB at conventional levels of fortification (40 mg/100 g), if fortified to target, provides 9.8 mg of vitamin C; 100 g of high-fortified CSB (90 mg/100 g) provides 43 mg of vitamin C. *If blended foods are considered the only source of vitamin C,* the cost of providing 10 mg of vitamin C with conventionally fortified CSB is 3.4 cents (range: 5 cents at 17 percent retention, 2.7 cents at 32 percent retention). With high-fortified CSB, 10 mg of vitamin C costs 0.79 cents. Highly fortified CSB is thus 4.3 times more cost-effective (range: 6.3 times at 17 percent retention, 3.4 times at 32 percent retention) as a delivery mechanism for vitamin C. A 30 g daily ration of blended food provides slightly less than 3 mg of vitamin C at conventional levels of fortification; at high levels, it would provide 12.9 mg, which would be sufficient to prevent scurvy. It would take 102 g of conventional CSB to provide 10 mg of vitamin C and 23 g of high-fortified CSB to provide the same amount. Recall, however, that 102 g of conventional CSB would also provide 388 calories, 18.7 g of protein, and additional quantities of other micronutrients, compared to only 87 calories, 4.2 g of protein, and comparably smaller amounts of other micronutrients in the highly fortified CSB.

Because of methodological problems in estimating the loss of vitamin C during cooking, two alternative calculations are presented here, with uniform rates of nutrient retention assumed for both conventional and highly fortified CSB at 30 and 60 percent. At a vitamin C retention rate of 30 percent, the cost of providing 10 mg of vitamin C in conventionally fortified CSB is 2.79 cents, and in highly fortified CSB it is 1.26 cents. A 30 g daily ration of conventionally fortified CSB would provide 3.6 mg of vitamin C; the same ration of highly fortified CSB would provide 8.1 mg. To provide 10 mg of vitamin C would require 83.3 g of conventional CSB and 37 g of highly fortified CSB.

At 60 percent retention, the cost of providing 10 mg of vitamin C would be 1.39 cents for conventional CSB and 0.63 cents for highly fortified CSB. The ration required to provide 10 mg of the vitamin would be 41.6 g of conventional or 18.5 g of highly fortified CSB. A 30 g ration of conventional CSB would provide 7.2 mg of vitamin C; a 30 g ration of highly fortified CSB would provide 16.2 mg.

However, we know that retention rates are higher when initial fortification levels are higher. If conventional CSB retains 30 percent of its fortificant and highly fortified CSB retains 60 percent, then providing 10 mg of vitamin C to an individual would cost 2.79 cents per day with conventional CSB and 0.63 cents per day with highly fortified CSB, suggesting that the highly fortified CSB may be as much as 4.4 times more cost effective as a vitamin C delivery mechanism

Note, though, that the reduction in quantity of ration implicit in this calculation would have serious implications for other nutrients contained in the blended food. Even though 18.5 g of highly fortified CSB would be sufficient to provide 10 mg of vitamin C under these assumptions, such a small ration would provide very low levels of the other macro- and micronutrients in the food. This food, although intended as a supplementary ration, is still *food*; it should not be treated as if it were simply a vitamin C pill.

Obviously, the rate of nutrient retention greatly affects the cost-effectiveness assessment. It is possible to generate a variety of alternative cost scenarios at various levels of retention. Although the best empirical information we have is used in the first set of estimates presented here, this information is limited because it comes from only two sites and from very few samples. Still, the conclusion is quite robust to alternative reasonable assumptions of nutrient retention. If only vitamin C consumption is considered and if blended foods are considered the only source, then highly fortified CSB is a more cost-effective delivery system than conventional CSB. If vitamin C consumption is considered in relation to the level of deficiency in the population, however, and other nutrient needs are also taken into account, this conclusion is not warranted. The results of the pilot suggest that even after transportation, storage, and cooking under the conditions observed in Haiti and Tanzania, there is still significant vitamin C left in the food. If simply delivering more vitamin C were the objective, then at reasonable estimates of nutrient retention, highly fortified CSB is a more cost effective mechanism for delivering vitamin C than conventional CSB. However, it is not more cost-effective for preventing scurvy.

Appropriateness of Blended Foods as a Strategy for Reducing the Risk of Vitamin C Deficiency

In most refugee situations, blended foods are not part of the general ration. Blended foods are provided in the general ration in situations where additional micronutrients are needed, for example, when access to local markets is cut off or when seasonal shortages occur. These foods are more often used as supplementary food in maternal and child health programs. When frank scurvy appears in refugee camps, distribution of blended foods is only one option considered; others include procurement of local foods containing vitamin C (a preferred strategy because such procurement can strengthen the local economy, the foods provide additional nutrients, and a quick response is possible) or provision of therapeutic doses through ascorbic acid tablet distribution. When blended foods are provided, WFP arranges to procure fortified blended foods from various suppliers (e.g., in Europe, South Africa) or to set up processing capacity for blended foods locally, using imported vitamin–mineral premixes. Some of these foods are fortified at higher levels than currently available P.L. 480 blended foods. The lag time for procuring blended foods from the United States if they have not routinely been provided is four to six months, too long for emergency response to an acute health problem. Although blended foods can forestall scurvy in at-risk camps that have no access to other sources of vitamin C-containing foods, different approaches are preferable under most circumstances.

Cost of Additional Fortification

The additional cost of raising the current fortification level of vitamin C from 40 to 90 mg/100 g is $6.33/MT of blended food (Table 3-1). These estimates are based on 1996 prices, which are considerably lower than prices from 1995; however, the price of vitamin C is expected to remain low for at least the next three years, due to the entry of China into the market as a producer of synthetic vitamin C (Ranum and Chomé, 1997). Since synthetic vitamin C is already purchased in bulk, there is no reason to expect that the price would fall further if the level of fortification were increased. The cost of a metric ton of blended food at current levels of fortification is $334.74 for CSB and $458.41 for WSB. The marginal cost of additional vitamin C fortification thus represents about 1.8 percent of the cost of CSB. The cost of vitamin C represents about one-third of total vitamin premix costs (see Appendix C).

For purposes of estimating the cost-effectiveness of increasing vitamin C fortification of blended foods, one must assume that the target fortification levels are reached consistently at the costs given. At present, this assumption is not correct. For cost-effectiveness analysis of the intervention to be meaningful we must first verify that the intervention is technically achievable. (Technical intervention to ensure consistency is addressed separately in Chapter 6 of this report.)

Ration Size

The SUSTAIN report states that the expected daily ration of fortified, blended food per person is 30 g. OMNI (1994) gives an expected ration of 40 g. Other reports say that the expected ration may be as high as 90 g per person per day or variable depending on need (T. Marchione, USAID, personal communication, June 1997). Planned distributions of CSB for fiscal year (FY) 1996 (USAID, 1996) are based on per-person daily rations ranging from 30 to 216 g. However, no information is available on quantities actually distributed or above all, on the reliability and consistency of distribution.

Clearly, if blended foods are provided at conventional levels of fortification but in higher amounts than the assumed 30 g per day ration, the conventionally-fortified ration could forestall scurvy and provide additional nutrients. A ration of about 102 g of conventionally fortified blended food would provide 10 mg of vitamin C, based on the pessimistic assumption of 24.5 percent nutrient retention after cooking. Of the highly fortified food, 23 g would provide 10 mg of vitamin C under the optimistic assumption of 48 percent nutrient retention. (If 30 percent nutrient retention is assumed for both, the necessary ration would be 83.3 g for the conventional and 30 g for the highly fortified food.) Providing a larger quantity of blended food has the considerable added advantage of supplying more of all the other macro- and micronutrients in the food. Since scurvy occurs mainly in cases of extreme need where refugees are entirely dependent on often inadequate relief rations, the other nutrients in the blends are likely to be just as necessary. For example, recent surveys in long-standing refugee camps in Kenya, Ethiopia, and Somalia where scurvy had previously been reported, showed prevalence of wasting (an indicator of protein-energy malnutrition [PEM]) of over 50 percent in Ethiopia, and 20 to 40 percent in Kenya. Camps in Kenya also had a prevalence of anemia of 75 to 85 percent (AAC/SCN, 1997). Further, if the ration is already closer to 100 g than to 30 g, current levels of fortification should be sufficient to provide the 10 mg of vitamin C required to prevent scurvy.

Cost-Effectiveness

Because of lack of information about the prevalence of vitamin C deficiency, an accurate estimate of the cost per case of scurvy averted is impossible. About 100,000 cases of scurvy have been reported over the past two decades or about 5,000 cases per year (Desenclos et al., 1989,). If the estimate is doubled and an incidence of 10,000 cases per year is assumed, and if all these cases could be averted simply by extra fortification, then the cost of averting a case of scurvy using extra fortification of CSB and WSB would be $158. Since at most 13 percent of refugees are reached by P.L. 480 blended foods (assuming a 30 g daily ration for a year), we may assume that at most only about 13 percent of scurvy cases could be averted using current allocations; if only 13 percent of the 10,000 cases per year could be averted through increased fortification, then the cost per case averted would be $1,223. At current prices, the cost of tripling the ration of conventionally fortified blended food from 30 to 90 g per person per day, an amount that would provide close to the 10 mg needed to prevent scurvy, would be an additional $7.45 per person per year, a total of $74,500 for 10,000 cases. Reported scurvy prevalence in high-risk camps ranges from 1 percent to as high as 45 percent for high risk subgroups (Magan et al., 1983, CDC, 1989; Desenclos et al., 1989; ACC/SCN, 1996). It would be virtually impossible to target rations narrowly only to potential scurvy sufferers inside the camps. If prevalence is about 20 percent, at most one fifth of the blended food would reach those who have scurvy or are likely to develop it, which would raise the cost per case averted or cured using conventionally fortified food to $37.25. If the prevalence were estimated at 10 percent (probably a more realistic estimate), the cost per case actually averted or cured would be $74.50. Thus even assuming that extra fortification could cure *all* cases of scurvy (using the estimate of 10,000 cases per year), tripling the conventional ration to high risk camps is more than twice as cost effective (cost-effectiveness ratio of 2.1) as fortifying the entire supply of blended food. If the proportion of cases that could be averted using extra fortification is the same as the proportion of refugees potentially covered by P.L. 480 blended food distribution (13 percent), then the ratio is 16.4: it would cost 16.4 times as much to avert a case of scurvy through extra fortification as through increasing the size of the conventional ration to beneficiaries in the target camps.

To avert 10,000 cases of scurvy per year would require a total of 109.5 MT of blended food at high levels of fortification, given a ration of 30 g per day for 365 days a year at a retention level of 48 percent. This amount represents 0.045 percent of the total blended food that would be available if the current amounts distributed were adjusted downward to account for the cost of extra vitamin C. At conventional levels of fortification, a ration of 102 g per day would be required, or 372.3 MT—about 0.15 percent of the total amount currently available. Since extra fortification raises the cost of blended foods by 1.8 percent, tripling the conventional ration for 10,000 recipients, which would reduce the amount available by only 0.14 percent, clearly is over 12.8 times more cost effective. If the triple ration were targeted by camp rather than individual suffering from scurvy and a prevalence rate of 10 percent were assumed, tripling the conventional ration would reduce the total amount of blended food available by 1.4 percent, which is still less than the 1.8 percent cost of fortifying the entire supply of blended food. Once again, this calculation considers only the benefit of providing vitamin C without taking account of the additional nutrients that would be provided in a triple ration.

Opportunity Cost

An important element of cost-effectiveness is opportunity cost. At current prices for blended foods and vitamin C, raising the level of fortification of CSB and WSB would cost $1,580,031, and would represent about 1.8 percent of the total cost of blended foods. If the budget for blended foods is fixed, raising the level of fortification of vitamin C in blended foods would reduce the total amount of blended food available by 186,499 metric tons, (1.8 percent; Ranum and Chomé, 1997). This quantity could provide a daily 30 g ration of conventionally fortified blended food to 425,797 people for a year and provide 114 kcal, 5–6 g of protein, and a wide range of micronutrients besides vitamin C to targeted vulnerable groups. Protein-energy malnutrition (PEM) and other micronutrient deficiencies (notably of vitamin A, iron, and iodine) are generally considered a higher public health priority than vitamin C deficiency, because of the larger numbers of people affected. This does not mean that the vitamin C currently provided in blended foods should be eliminated. There are rare cases in which refugees are entirely dependent on donated rations, with no possibility of trading with the outside or of producing their own food. In these cases, the vitamin C in blended food is necessary because it may well be the sole source.

Higher fortification of U.S.-provided blended foods may not be the most efficient or cost-effective of these alternatives. Other approaches to improving vitamin C nutrition in refugee camps are likely to be more cost-effective. For instance, use of local food sources rich in vitamin C benefits the local economy and provides additional nutrients in the foods. Local foods can be obtained quickly, to respond to the need for vitamin C in a timely way. Alternative approaches for the prevention of scurvy should be explored in situations where the availability of vitamin C-rich foods is low.

Iron Objective

A secondary argument for providing additional vitamin C in blended food is that it enhances the absorption of iron; thus, it might be possible to reduce the amount of iron in blended food if additional vitamin C were provided. The current cost of fortifying blended foods with iron is $1.61/MT. If this level could be cut by half with the addition of vitamin C at proposed levels (which is probably an overestimate), the cost of iron fortification per metric ton would be reduced by 80 cents, whereas the cost of the additional vitamin C would be $6.33. Thus, the net effect of improving iron absorption through the addition of vitamin C would be an additional cost of $5.52 per metric ton; obviously, adding vitamin C is not a cost-effective strategy for improving the absorption of iron from blended foods.

Although there are many approaches that could be considered to improve iron intake, this substantial difference in cost-effectiveness and the uncertainty about the stability of vitamin C make it unlikely that further comparisons would alter this conclusion. In fact, it may be better to replace the present form of iron used in blended foods with another form, since the present form is poorly absorbed and reduces vitamin C retention. A more complete cost-effectiveness analysis should consider other forms of iron, but this is beyond the scope of the committee's assignment. It seems most unlikely that such analysis would result in recommending an increase in vitamin C fortification to improve iron absorption.

4

Results of the Vitamin C Pilot Program

As directed by Congress, the U.S. Agency for International Development (USAID) developed and implemented a pilot program to produce and provide blended food aid commodities with enhanced levels of vitamin C fortification to at least two field sites. USAID implemented a cooperative agreement with the organization SUSTAIN (Sharing United States Technology to Aid in the Improvement of Nutrition) to implement the pilot program so that it would represent closely ordinary food aid operations from procurement through distribution at field sites. SUSTAIN's primary responsibilities included (1) monitoring and statistically analyzing the variability in vitamin C content of fortified blends at the manufacturing site and estimating the production costs; (2) monitoring vitamin C losses during shipping, storage, and distribution; (3) estimating vitamin C losses during food preparation; and (4) collecting dietary information to estimate the contribution of the commodity to the recipients' total daily vitamin C intake. This chapter summarizes the pilot program implemented by SUSTAIN and outlines its major findings.

SUMMARY OF THE PILOT PROGRAM

SUSTAIN developed two vitamin premixes. One provided the standard level of vitamin C fortification of 40 mg/100 g of dry blended cereal when added at the rate of 908 g per metric ton (MT). The other premix provided vitamin C fortification at the level of 90 mg/100 g of dry blended cereals when added at the rate of 1,363 g/MT. Contracts for production of the pilot procurements were awarded to the lowest bidder using standard USDA–CCC (U.S. Department of Agriculture, Commodity Credit Corporation) procurement procedures. Two production plants were selected to prepare the fortified cereals:

plant A produced 500 MT of corn–soy blend (CSB) with high vitamin C and 500 MT of CSB with conventional levels of vitamin C; and plant B made 240 MT of conventionally fortified wheat–soy blend (WSB) followed by 240 MT of WSB with high vitamin C. Special markings were printed on the bags of these pilot production runs to facilitate finding the bags for sampling when they reached their distribution locations.

Countries chosen by the USAID's Office of Food for Peace and SUSTAIN for the pilot program were Haiti for WSB, a regular development type of food aid program and Tanzania for CSB, an emergency feeding situation. The primary criteria for site selection were that at least one country food aid program had to be chosen where scurvy had been reported in past camp feeding situations and one program where significant iron deficiency has been reported. Although there have been no reports of scurvy emanating from Tanzania to date, its location in the greater Horn of Africa where numerous cases of scurvy have been reported and the emergency feeding situation in the camps there indicated a very high risk situation.

Determination of Vitamin C Uniformity in Commodities at Manufacture

Based on recommendations from the statistical subgroup of SUSTAIN's advisory panel, 48 samples of each run were collected. Sample collection was spread evenly over a two- to three-day run time. Ten of these samples were duplicated for use as blind analytical checks. A SUSTAIN representative, with the assistance of the USDA Feed Grain Inspection Service (FGIS) inspector and plant Quality Control (QC) staff, collected samples from each production run. Determination of whether a pilot production run was worthy of continued study was based on the following criteria: (1) the production was within control limits by normal standards of statistical quality control as applied by the U.S. food industry and (2) the variance in production was small enough to detect a 20 percent drop in ascorbic acid content at a 95 percent confidence level.

After initial results indicated uniformity problems in the fortification of CSB, USAID and the SUSTAIN Vitamin C Advisory Panel agreed that each of the seven plants that had been awarded CSB and WSB production contracts should be sampled to assess the extent of the problem. Five of the seven plants were sampled; 4 of the 5 CSB manufacturing plants and one of the two WSB manufacturing plants. The remaining two plants were not in production during the sampling period. Because the vitamin C content of the special CSB produced in plant A did not meet its criteria of acceptability for further study, SUSTAIN planned to postpone field testing of CSB in Tanzania indefinitely. However, in its preliminary report on the pilot program (IOM, 1996), the Institute of Medicine Committee on International Nutrition recommended to SUSTAIN that retrieval and analysis of samples of CSB delivered to Tanzania would be of value for two reasons: (1) to determine if vitamin C remained in the samples even though the mean concentration could not be specified precisely and (2) to provide information on the mean vitamin C content and its variability in field samples that would be needed to examine cost-effectiveness. In this situation, locating the coded bags to obtain paired samples for analysis would be more critical.

Because of concern over the variability in vitamin C content of CSB shipped to Tanzania, another production lot of CSB, which had been shipped to India from a plant that met SUSTAIN's criteria for uniformity, was identified for field testing of cooking losses. This material contained only the standard level of 40 mg of vitamin C per 100 g of dry commodity.

Determination of Vitamin C Stability from Manufacture to Distribution Sites

The stability of vitamin C was to be assessed by the following independent methods:

• Analysis of mean levels and variation of vitamin C content at production of the CSB and WSB compared to the same lot of product just prior to food preparation in the recipient country.

• Analysis of paired samples of specially marked bags: Once the specially marked sampled bags were located in the field and sampled, their vitamin C content was compared to the vitamin C content found in the same bags during production.

• Using niacin as a marker of vitamin fortification: Niacin, which is included in the vitamin premix for fortification of CSB and WSB, is considered a highly stable vitamin and is not likely to show a decrease during storage and transport. Since the vitamin premix has a uniform ratio of niacin to vitamin C, a change in this ratio would reflect a loss of vitamin C. Because of a number of limitations associated with this method, it was intended to be used only if the other two methods failed due to inadequate data. Ultimately, it was not used as a measure of vitamin C retention.

Time intervals from production to distribution site samplings represented transport and storage time and were seven months for CSB sampled in Tanzania, nine months for WSB sampled in Haiti (Box 4-1 and 4-2), and five months for CSB sampled in India.

Box 4-1. Schedule of the CSB Special Procurement from Production to
Distribution in the Refugee Camps of Western Tanzania

Date	Event
06/24/96–06/28/96	Production at Plant A, Wisconsin, USA (500 MT)
	Production sampling by SUSTAIN
08/10/96–08/20/96	Shipment from New Orleans, Louisiana
10/11/96	Arrival in Dar-es-Salaam, Tanzania
10/26/96	Discharge at Dar-es-Salaam in warehouse at port (495 MT was received by WFP)
10/25/96 and 10/29/96	Transport to Isaka, Cargo Center
11/4/96	Departure from Isaka to Ngara for the first consignment
11/25/96	Second consignment
	Distribution in Ngara region at a rate of 105 MT/week (for the general distribution) + Special Feeding Programs
	A total of 350 MT of this procurement was distributed in the Ngara region.
12/9/96	Last day of distribution from this special procurement (21.854 MT remaining, this was not enough for one week's worth distribution). This was distributed when a new procurement of blended food was delivered.
01/17/97–01/23/97	Sampling in the camps by SUSTAIN

SOURCE: Ranum and Chomé, 1997.

Box 4-2. Schedule of the WSB Special Procurement from Production to
Distribution in Haiti

Date	Event
07/08/96–07/12/96	Production at plant B, Missouri (480 MT)
	Production sampling by SUSTAIN
07/30/96	Shipment from Lake Charles, Louisiana, to Haiti
08/12/96	Arrival in Port-au-Prince, Haiti
10/14/96	Transport from port to warehouse (19,146 bags were counted at reception, equivalent to 479 MT)
12/09/96	First day of special procurement distribution to MCH and OCF centers. Distribution to the different centers is done on a continuous basis. Each center receives a delivery every three months.
3/11/97–3/21/97	Sampling in Haiti by SUSTAIN
6/01/97	Completion of distribution to the centers
9/01/97	Approximate date when the last of the special procurement will be distributed to the mothers at the center level

SOURCE: Ranum and Chomé, 1997.

Vitamin C Retention During Food Preparation

Food preparation studies were conducted in both Haiti and Tanzania. The purpose of data collection on food preparation was to determine the extent to which vitamin C is lost as a result of typical preparation techniques. Objectives were (1) to document the food preparation methods used by beneficiaries of food aid in two feeding programs and (2) to sample prepared foods from several beneficiary households for vitamin C analysis. Preliminary observations had shown that in Haiti the most commonly prepared WSB dishes were gruel, and dumplings cooked in a vegetable broth. In the Tanzanian refugee camps the most commonly prepared CSB dishes were gruel and *ugali* (a Swahili word referring to a stiff porridge traditionally prepared with fermented cassava). Gruel was the most commonly prepared food for both CSB and WSB, accounting for 24 out of 39 samples. Details of the complete methodology used can be found in Ranum and Chomé (1997) and cooking loss data are summarized in Table 4-1.

TABLE 4-1. Summary of Vitamin C Retention After Cooking

Commodity	Level of Vitamin C	Cooking Method	Vitamin C in CSB/WSB Prior to Cooking Dry Basis (mg/100g)	% Retention (95% Confidence Interval)[a]
CSB	Conventional	Gruel (n = 9)	24–40	9.6% (4.3%–21.5%)
CSB[b]	Conventional	Ugali (n = 1)	27	48.1% (—)
CSB	High	Gruel (n = 7)	97–177	55.1% (47.6%–63.9%)
CSB	High	Ugali (n = 4)	104–177	51.3% (31.4%–84.1%)
WSB	Conventional	Gruel (n = 3)	38–41	27.4% (22.0%–34.2%)
WSB	Conventional	Dumplings (n = 4)	38–43	16.4% (10.1%–26.7%)
WSB	High	Gruel (n = 5)	73–88	30.9% (24.5%–38.9%)
WSB	High	Dumplings (n = 5)	71–92	26.5% (12.4%–56.5%)

[a] Confidence intervals were obtained from raw data (not adjusted for initial level of vitamin C).
[b] Only one preparation of ugali made from CSB sampled.

SOURCE: Ranum and Chomé, 1997.

MAJOR FINDINGS OF THE PILOT PROGRAM

• **Uniformity of vitamin C in commodities at manufacturing site.** Following the initial sampling of CSB, which indicated poor uniformity of product, the consensus was that each of the seven CSB and WSB plants that were awarded production contracts should be sampled. Five of seven plants were sampled, and results indicated that only two of the five plants—one batch processor and one continuous processor—met contract specifications most of the time (>90 percent). Two of the other plants (both utilizing a continuous process) were outside specifications more than 50 percent of the time.

• **Stability of vitamin C from manufacture to points of distribution.** The vitamin C stability component of the study did not include data from Tanzania because the CSB pilot production sent to Tanzania was not sufficiently uniform to allow for efficient testing. The WSB sent to Haiti with conventional levels of added vitamin C showed a small but statistically significant loss of 13 percent. The WSB sent to Haiti with the high level of vitamin C, and the CSB shipped to India with conventional levels of vitamin C both showed essentially 100 percent retention of added vitamin C. Results from comparison of mean levels and comparison of paired samples in specially marked bags were very similar.

• **Vitamin C retention during food preparation.** Results from these studies showed large losses of vitamin C in both CSB and WSB in prepared food made from these commodities (Tables 4-2 and 4-3). The magnitude of this loss for CSB was inversely proportional to concentration: the higher the level of the vitamin in the dry commodity before cooking, the greater was the retention. Retention of the conventional level of added vitamin C was 17–32 percent in CSB and 27 percent for WSB gruel samples. At the high level of added vitamin C, the retention was 44–74 percent for CSB and an average of 32 percent for WSB. Five out of nine gruel samples, made from CSB with the conventional level of vitamin C, showed vitamin C content to be below the level of detection of 1 mg/100 g.

• **Analysis of vitamin C cost.** The best cost estimate of adding vitamin C to CSB and WSB manufacturer, if the proposed change were instituted today, is $6.33/MT. Based on Fiscal Year 1996 purchases, this would have meant spending an additional $1,580,000 per year. It is important to note that the price of ethyl cellulose-coated vitamin C varies depending primarily on the price of ascorbic acid. The current base price of ascorbic acid is at an all time low, $5–$7/kg in 1997 (Ranum and Chomé, 1997). In 1995 the actual prices paid for ascorbic acid by a large vitamin premix manufacturer ranged from $13.40 to $15.75/kg.

TABLE 4-2. Tanzania Samples—CSB Food Preparations, Vitamin C Data

Sample Type	Moisture in CSB Before Cooking (% by wt.) (a)	Moisture in Food Mixture After Cooking (% by wt.) (b)	Vitamin C in CSB Before Cooking Wet Basis (mg/100 g) (c)	Vitamin C in CSB Before Cooking Dry Basis (mg/100 g) (d) [c/(100-a)]x100	Vitamin C in Food Mixture After Cooking, Wet Basis (mg/100 g) (e)	Vitamin C in Food Mixture After Cooking, Dry Basis (mg/199 g) (f) [e/(100-b)]x100	Vitamin C Retention, Dry Basis (%) (g) (f/d) x 100	Time in Water Before Cooking (min:sec)	Time of Cooking (min:sec)
High C									
gruel	9.57	92.6	95	105	4	54	51	7	11
gruel	9.63	88.4	88	97	5	43	44	3	6
gruel	9.74	88.5	96	106	6	52	49	3	8
Average (n = 3)	9.65	89.8	93	103	5	50	48	4.3	8.3
SD	0.09	2.4	4	5	1	6	4	2.3	2.5
gruel	9.52	89.1	160	177	14	128	73	2	15
gruel	9.57	87.7	160	177	16	130	74	0:45	16
gruel	9.55	86.4	160	177	13	96	54	0	29
Average (n = 3)	9.55	87.7	160	177	14	118	67	0:55	20
SD	0.03	1.4	0	0	2	19	11	1:0	7:48
therap.gruel	9.19	75	68	75	9	36	48	5:30	2.30
ugali	9.66	51.4	94	104	18	37	36	0	7
ugali	9.71	61.0	96	106	15	38	36	0	6
ugali	9.55	57.4	140	155	49	115	74	0	3:37
ugali	9.53	56.0	160	177	57	130	73	0	4
Average (n =4)	9.61	56.5	122.5	135.5	34.8	80	54.8	0	5
SD	0.09	40	32.8	36.4	21.4	49.5	21.7	0	2

continued

TABLE 4-2. *Continued*

Sample Type (a)	Moisture in CSB Before Cooking (% by wt.) (a)	Moisture in Food Mixture After Cooking (% by wt.) (b)	Vitamin C in CSB Before Cooking Wet Basis (mg/100 g) (c)	Vitamin C in CSB Before Cooking Dry Basis (mg/100 g) (d) [c/(100-a)]x100	Vitamin C in Food Mixture After Cooking, Wet Basis (mg/100 g) (e)	Vitamin C in Food Mixture After Cooking, Dry Basis (mg/199 g) (f) [e/(100-b)]x100	Vitamin C Retention, Dry Basis (%) (g) (f/d)x100	Time in Water Before Cooking (min:sec)	Time of Cooking (min:sec)
Conventional C									
gruel	9.46	86.5	36	40	BLD[a]	<7	<19	NA	9:26
gruel	9.45	85.0	23	25	BLD	<7	<26	NA	8:32
gruel	9.43	89.7	22	24	BLD	<10	<40	NA	8:00
gruel	9.39	89.9	28	31	1	10	32	NA	10:44
gruel	9.33	92.0	34	37	BLD	<13	<33	NA	8:30
gruel	9.57	86.6	27	30	2	15	50	3	20
gruel	9.57	81.4	33	36	2	11	29	4	15
gruel	9.50	90.7	25	28	1	11	39	5	6
soup[b]	9.63	80.9	29	32	BLD	<5	<16	12	12
Average	9.48	87.0	29	32	1	5 to 10	17 to 32	19	11
SD (n = 9)	0.10	4.0	5	5	0 to 1	3 to 6	11 to 21	6	4
ugali	9.62	48.1	24	27	7	13	51	5	5
fried cake	9.81	39.8	28	31	1	2	5	5	5

NOTE: Vitamin C level of detection is 1 mg/100 g. (Entries in column (e) that read BLD 0–1 mg/100 g of vitamin C lead to corresponding ranges in columns (f) and (g).); SD = standard deviation ; wt = weight.

[a] BLD = Below level of detection.
[b] Soup with 500 g tomato, 20 g onion, 110 g oil.

SOURCE: Ranum and Chomé, 1997.

TABLE 4-3. Haiti Samples—WSB Food Preparations Vitamin C Data

Sample Type	Moisture in WSB Before Cooking (% by wt.) (a)	Moisture in Food Mixture After Cooking (% by wt.) (b)	Vitamin C in WSB Before Cooking Wet Basis (mg/100 g) (c)	Vitamin C in WSB Before Cooking Dry Basis (mg/100 g) (d) [c/(100-a)]x100	Vitamin C in Food Mixture After Cooking, Wet Basis (mg/100 g) (e)	Vitamin C in Food Mixture After Cooking, Dry Basis (mg/100 g) (f) [e/(100-b)]x100	Vitamin C Retention, Dry Basis (%) (g) (f/d)x100	Time in Water Before Cooking (min:sec)	Time of Cooking (min:sec)
High C									
gruel	7.67	79.6	67	73	4	20	27	6:00	15:00
gruel	7.82	73.9	73	79	7	27	34	10:30	18:32
gruel	7.73	79.5	79	86	6	29	34	3:34	21:00
gruel	7.61	77.7	81	88	8	36	41	14:00	17:00
gruel	7.70	76.4	72	78	4	17	22	6:00	19:00
Average (n = 5)	7.71	77.4	74	81	6	26	32	8	18
SD (n = 5)	0.08	2.4	6	6	2	8	7	4	2
dumplings	7.79	62.7	76	82	9	24	29	13:00	24:00
dumplings	7.64	56.3	85	92	22	50	55	13:00	13:00
dumplings	7.62	61.8	66	71	2	5	7	8:00	18:00
dumplings	7.52	64.4	83	90	14	39	44	14:00	24:00
dumplings	7.78	57.7	82	89	11	26	29	7:00	24:22
Average (n = 5)	7.67	60.6	78	85	12	29	33	11	21
SD (n = 5)	0.11	3.4	8	8	7	17	18	3	6

continued

TABLE 4-3. *Continued*

Sample Type	Moisture in WSB Before Cooking (% by wt.) (a)	Moisture in Food Mixture After Cooking (% by wt.) (b)	Vitamin C in WSB Before Cooking Wet Basis (mg/100 g) (c)	Vitamin C in WSB Before Cooking Dry Basis (mg/100 g) (d) [c/(100-a)]x100	Vitamin C in Food Mixture After Cooking, Wet Basis (mg/100 g) (e)	Vitamin C in Food Mixture After Cooking, Dry Basis (mg/100 g) (f) [e/(100-b)]x100	Vitamin C Retention, Dry Basis (%) (g) (f/d)x100	Time in Water Before Cooking (min:sec)	Time of Cooking (min:sec)
Conventional C									
gruel	7.55	81.0	38	41	2	11	26	10:30	13:00
gruel	7.71	83.0	35	38	2	12	31	10:50	25:25
gruel	7.60	79.9	38	41	2	10	24	10:00	25:35
Average (n = 3)	7.62	81.3	37	40	2	11	27	10	21
SD (n = 3)	0.08	1.6	2	2	0	1	4	0	7
dumplings	7.60	61.0	40	43	5	13	30	8:00	13:00
dumplings	7.98	62.9	35	38	2	5	14	11:00	18:00
dumplings	7.43	59.9	37	40	2	5	12	10:00	19:00
dumplings	7.68	47.5	38	41	3	6	14	10:10	8:34
Average (n = 4)	7.67	57.8	38	41	3	7	18	10	15
SD (n = 4)	0.23	7.0	2	2	1	4	8	1	5

SOURCE: Ranum and Chomé, 1997.

5

Critique of the Pilot Program

UNIFORMITY OF BLENDED COMMODITIES

Four of the six U.S. plants producing corn–soy blend (CSB) were assessed to determine plant performance and conformity to good manufacturing practices (GMPs). Attainment of target fortification levels for vitamin C in CSB requires understanding the inherent capability of both the dosing-metering unit operation and the blending equipment. CSB is made by a continuous process in which very low percentages of minor ingredients are metered into a large bulk stream. In this type of mixing, there is the distinct possibility that minor ingredients may remain segregated or unmixed. Failure to achieve uniform dispersion in a continuous process is a common food processing concern.

The sampling analysis submitted by SUSTAIN (Sharing United States Technology to Aid in the Improvement of Nutrition) provides ample evidence of a problem in the uniformity of finished CSB product. Analytical sampling for vitamin C content showed significant failure to achieve consistent enrichment levels of 40 mg or 90 mg per 100 g of commodity. Extensive plant-to-plant variability was observed, supporting the notion that plants encountered technical challenges in metering and blending the vitamin premix. SUSTAIN data indicated that two plants (C and E) were more capable than plants A and D in achieving acceptable compliance levels. It should be noted that none of the four plants consistently achieved target fortification levels of vitamin C at either doseage.

Wheat–soy blend (WSB) is prepared in a batch system whereby all ingredients are mixed simultaneously. It is easier to obtain homogeneous mixing with a batch process than with a continuous process, but batch processing is suitable for only relatively small amounts of product. WSB production on a batch system was sampled at one of the two U.S. manufacturing sites: plant B was capable of consistently achieving the conventional target of 40 mg/100 g

47

but operated below target for the higher vitamin C level. Even though the batch process delivered the best performance, it is recognized that WSB represents only a small fraction of total blended products distributed by the Public Law (P.L.) 480 Title II program.

CAPABILITY OF THE PRODUCTION PROCESS TO MEET PRODUCT SPECIFICATIONS

The target vitamin C values for conventional and higher levels of fortification are 40 and 90 mg per 100 g, respectively. Many factors combine to produce variation in the measured values of vitamin C in samples from production runs. When processes are *in control,* vitamin C is approximately normally distributed. Consequently, 99.7 percent of the values will be within 3 S.D. (standard deviations) of the mean. When making control charts, extremes such as the mean ±3 S.D., are called the upper and lower control limits (UCL and LCL).

Specifications (SPECS) refer to the limits that define acceptable product. Generally these are determined by the customer, and any product outside these limits is reprocessed or discarded. Appropriate SPECS depend on the product and the property being measured. For example, a 12-ounce soft drink product might have a lower SPEC only for volume (if the can contains less than 12 ounces the customer has not received what has been paid for, but excess product is acceptable). On the other hand, the sugar content would have upper and lower SPECS; a drink that is either too sweet or not sweet enough is unacceptable. For some products an 80 percent rule is used: a product that contains at least 80 percent of the quantity advertised is acceptable. It is important to note that SPECS refer to the acceptability of a product, not to the mean and standard deviation of the process that yields the product. Very often, a target value is used, which is in the middle of the upper and lower SPECS. It is also important to note that under current USDA–CCC procurement procedures for P.L. 480 Title II blended commodities that specifications are written for the manufacturing process (e.g. how much of the nutrient must be added during manufacture), not on the nutrient content of the final product.

Process capability refers to measures that express how well the production process satisfies the SPECS. These measures take several forms but generally can be translated into the proportion of product that is unacceptable. There are two ways to ensure that this proportion is small: (1) the process mean should be close to the target value, and (2) the standard deviation of the process should be small. In many processes, the first is relatively easy to achieve by adjusting a component. For example, if the process mean for vitamin C in conventional CSB is 27 mg/100 g, the equipment should be adjusted to add approximately 50 percent more premix in order to achieve the desired level of 40 mg/100 g.

Reducing the standard deviation is often a more complex job, involving the identification and control of sources of process variation.

The process capability index (Cp) compares the UCL and LCL to the SPECS. Specifically, Cp is the ratio of the difference between the upper and lower SPECs divided by the difference between the UCL and the LCL. Implicit in the use of this measure is the assumption that the process mean is either on target or can easily be moved there. If the Cp is 1.0, the two sets of limits coincide and the proportion of unacceptable product is the proportion falling above or below 3 S.D. from the mean (i.e., 100 percent–99.7 percent, or 0.3 percent). In some industries, a Cp of 1.33 or better is required to become a qualified supplier, whereas 2.00 is required to be a preferred or long-term supplier.

Samples collected by SUSTAIN of production runs at four or five CSB manufacturing plants and one of two WSB manufacturing plants were analyzed for both reduced and oxidized forms of vitamin C. A commercial statistical software program was used to analyze this data on production samples. This program, in addition to calculating upper and lower control limits and a number of descriptive statistics, also calculates the Cp (Ranum and Chomé, 1997). For CSB the Cp values ranged from 0.26 to 0.90 when the SPECs were set at 29–55 mg/100 g for conventional fortification and 65–120 mg/100 g for the high level of vitamin C. The Cp's were 0.20 and 0.85 for the two WSB productions in the same plant. Although these SPECs are somewhat arbitrary, the resulting calculations indicate that improvements are needed. For conventional CSB with a mean vitamin C content of 27.0 mg/100 g, 55 percent of the product is below the lower SPEC and 4 percent is above. It is also important to note that in three of the seven runs examined, an outlier was discarded. For a sample size of approximately 50 samples per run, this amounts to 2 percent, which indicates that these processes are not in control. This lack of control will simultaneously affect the content of other vitamins and minerals added to the CSB since both the vitamin and the mineral premixes are metered in at very low quantities.

STABILITY OF VITAMIN C DURING TRANSPORT AND STORAGE

The SUSTAIN report (Ranum and Chomé, 1997) notes that there were minimal losses of vitamin C in shipping, transport, and storage of CSB shipped to India and WSB to Haiti. The WSB (conventional vitamin C) loss was 13 percent (p < .01). However, the high vitamin C WSB shipped to Haiti and the conventional vitamin C CSB shipped to India had no losses (retention ~100 percent). Shipping, transport, and storage time for shipments to Haiti was nine months (see Box 4-2) and for India, five months. No data are available on transport and storage losses for shipments to Tanzania because of problems in uniformity encountered in the production of fortified CSB sent there. However, the time from production to distribution was seven months (see Box 4-1). The results of the pilot study, therefore, indicate that vitamin C is stable under the conditions encountered in shipping, transport, and storage.

VITAMIN C COOKING LOSSES

Limited numbers of samples were collected for vitamin C retention studies in prepared foods made with CSB and WSB.

Haiti—WSB

The most complete set of information on vitamin C retention during food preparation was provided for WSB foods in Haiti. The numbers of samples tested for the high and the conventional fortification levels were not the same (Table 5-1): for the high level, five gruel and five dumpling samples were collected; for the conventional level, three gruel and four dumpling samples. This is a very small sample for testing the hypothesis that vitamin C is retained in cooked foods.

TABLE 5-1. Summary of Food Preparation Samples Collected in Selected Countries

WSB, Haiti	No. of Samples	CSB, Tanzania	No. of Samples
High vitamin C		High vitamin C	
gruel	5	gruel	7
dumplings	5	ugali	4
Conventional vitamin C		Conventional vitamin C	
gruel	3	gruel	9
dumplings	4	ugali	1
		fried cake	1

SOURCE: Ranum and Chomé, 1997.

Means and standard deviations (S. D.) of vitamin C retention in WSB foods shipped to Haiti are fairly consistent (high C level: 32 ± 7 percent was retained in gruel and 33 ± 18 percent in dumplings; conventional C level: 27 ± 4 percent was retained in gruel and 18 ± 8 percent in dumplings, see Table 4-3). These results suggest that a smaller percentage of total vitamin C is retained at the conventional level of fortification. This is expected because vitamin C is less stable in dilute solutions than in more concentrated ones, particularly at the neutral pH of these foods (Hornig and Moser, 1981; Erdman and Klein, 1982). However, the overall average of ~27.5 percent retention in both gruel and dumplings is lower than expected or desirable. The average amount of vitamin

C in the cooked foods ranges from 2 to 6 mg per 100 g of gruel, and 3 to 12 mg per 100 g of dumplings. The intake of vitamin C from a serving of gruel (estimated as 150 g) would be greater than from a serving of dumplings (estimated at 40 g).

Differences in retention between dumplings and gruel may be attributed to the fact that gruel absorbs all of the cooking water, including any vitamin C that is dissolved during the soaking process. When dumplings are cooked, some vitamin C may be leached into the cooking liquid, but would ultimately be consumed. In this case, the total amounts of vitamin C retained in the two types of cooked foods may be similar, although product analysis indicates different amounts present.

Tanzania—CSB

For Tanzania, the sampling was more limited than Haiti. There were seven gruel and four ugali samples for the high C level and nine gruel, one ugali, and one fried cake for the conventional C level. Complete preparation information is not available for all the samples because of a problem with the scales when data were collected. Recipes and cooking times were not as well documented in Tanzania as in Haiti.

Data for CSB products from Tanzania are complicated by the inconsistent vitamin C content of the CSB produced by plant A. Because of this, CSB with the high fortification level of vitamin C was stratified into four groups (68, 93, 140, and 160 mg per 100 g of CSB). This further complicates interpretation of the data. Data are presented only for products prepared with 93 or 160 mg of product (see Table 4-2).

CSB gruel in Tanzania had higher moisture content (90 percent) than WSB gruel in Haiti (80 percent). Thus, losses would be expected to be higher in the more dilute gruel. This was true for the conventional-C CSB gruel (initial content 22 ± 5 mg/100 g), where retention was below detectable amounts of vitamin C for almost all nine gruel samples. Therefore, the data for retention, which were estimated as 17–32 percent, are questionable.

For the high-C CSB gruel, the three samples initially containing ~100 mg/100 g of CSB retained 48 percent of the vitamin C. In samples with an initial content of 177 mg/100 g, ~67 percent of the vitamin C was retained. On average, gruel contained 4–16 mg/100 g when made with any of the higher levels of vitamin C. Less than 1 mg/100 g remained in the conventional C gruel. This is in line with the theory that vitamin C is more stable in more concentrated solutions.

General Comments

Sample handling after cooking may have been less than optimal. The samples were placed in 4-ounce containers, which were put into insulated containers with frozen ice packs and moved to frozen storage approximately eight hours later. The cooler and freezer temperatures were monitored. However, it is both possible and likely that some vitamin C was lost in the initial cooling phase, particularly in the lower vitamin C samples. Thus, the vitamin C content of some or all of the analyzed samples of prepared foods may actually have been higher than reported. This suggests the need for follow-up of changes in vitamin C content during the immediate postcooking period.

Cooking procedures used in the field (in both Tanzania and Haiti) included soaking steps followed by heating. Cooking times were ~20–30 minutes, including soaking. Both CSB and WSB are processed to allow briefer cooking periods, and in situations of limited fuel this would be very important. Shorter heating periods could result in greater vitamin C retention because the primary cause of loss is heating.

In theory, 30 g of the WSB or CSB fortified at the conventional level of 40 mg/100 g or the high level of 90 mg/100 g would provide 12 or 27 mg of ascorbic acid, respectively if there were no cooking losses. If ~30 percent retention is assumed for WSB gruel, the intake would be 3.6 or 11.4 mg. Similarly, for conventional-level CSB gruel, retention was estimated at 30 percent, so intake would be 3.6 mg. At the high levels (starting material >90 mg/100 g), between 13.5 and 18 mg could be provided. If the intake of vitamin C was actually above 10 mg per day, this would be sufficient to prevent scurvy.

6

Conclusions and Recommendations

CONCLUSIONS

Programmatic approaches to provide displaced populations with adequate vitamin C must address two possible situations: (1) treatment of populations in which scurvy exists, and (2) provision of sufficient amounts of vitamin C to prevent scurvy in populations that are not currently deficient but are dependent to some degree on donated food commodities. The provision of sufficient amounts of vitamin C for other physiological purposes, such as maintenance of saturated tissue levels of ascorbic acid and enhancement of immune responses, was considered. However, these functions are less well documented, and appropriate levels to achieve such benefits are not known but are assumed to be much higher than those necessary for scurvy prevention. Thus, the committee concluded that assigning a priority to the addition of vitamin C in emergency feeding situations based on these roles, is not appropriate. The committee also estimated that adding additional vitamin C is not a cost-effective strategy for increasing the amount of iron absorbed from blended foods.

Assessment of Vitamin C Status and Risk of Deficiency

As a first step in determining the appropriate means of delivering vitamin C, it is necessary to assess the current situation of the population and the likelihood of future deficiency. Issues to be considered are (1) the current prevalence of scurvy, based on a specific case definition (e.g., presence of hemorrhagic skin lesions: or in nonedentulous children and adults, swollen, hemorrhagic gums, and either joint pain or muscle tenderness) and (2) access to vitamin C-containing foods.

Access to vitamin C-containing foods depends on the ability of the population to purchase food or engage in trade, the presence of local markets, and the availability of vitamin C-containing foods in these markets or the ability of food donors to purchase and provide such foods. Because of seasonal variation in the availability of these foods and dynamic changes in the market situation, periodic assessments are needed. It is extremely unlikely that biochemical assessment of vitamin C status will be feasible in most field situations, although this might be of interest for research purposes.

Ideally, systematic evaluation of the situation with regard to vitamin C should be included in the initial and subsequent periodic assessments of a population's general nutrition and health condition. It would be useful for international agencies and nongovernmental organizations to achieve some consensus on how this assessment might be accomplished and interpreted.

In any situation where more than 0.1 percent of individuals are found to have clinical scurvy, therapeutic interventions should be initiated as quickly as possible. Because the appearance of any cases of scurvy is likely to indicate that the entire population is deficient to some degree, therapeutic approaches might be considered for all members of the population until adequate preventive measures are in place. Moreover, since there is generally a lag of two to three months between the onset of low vitamin C intake and the first appearance of clinical signs of scurvy, it can be assumed that if any scurvy is present in a population at the initial assessment, the incidence of new disease is likely to increase progressively unless the population has access to local food sources of vitamin C or other preventive measures are introduced.

Occurrence of Scurvy

There is evidence of scurvy outbreaks among refugee populations entirely dependent on emergency relief rations that provide less than 2 mg of vitamin C per day per person. The greatest number of outbreaks occurred in the 1980s in Somalia. Only four outbreaks have been reported since January 1994, when the World Food Programme (WFP) and the United Nations High Commissioner for Refugees (UNHCR) adopted a policy of providing fortified blended foods to populations wholly dependent on food aid, in an effort to preempt any micronutrient deficiencies. One outbreak occurred among Rwandan refugees in eastern Zaire in the spring of 1994 prior to the time at which the newly adopted food aid plan could be implemented. Recurring mild outbreaks of scurvy were reported among Bhutanese refugees in Nepal in 1994, 1995, and 1996, and moderate outbreaks were reported among Somali refugees in the Dadaab camp in Kenya in 1994 and 1996. However, the scurvy outbreaks in the Dadaab camp did not appear to be related to the presence or abscence of fortified, blended foods in the diet. Thus, the need for higher vitamin C fortification of corn–soy blend (CSB) and wheat–soy blend (WSB) would be sporadic and apparently localized.

Treatment of Scurvy

Scurvy is best treated by administering large daily doses of vitamin C, which are typically provided as pharmaceutical preparations available in many dosages. Single doses on alternate day schedules would be needed. Response times depend on the extent of depletion. Because young children are often unable to swallow pills, special liquid or powdered preparations may be necessary, or vitamin C tablets would have to be manipulated in the household. For example, vitamin C tablets can be crushed and added to a prepared food or drink. However, because of the lability of ascorbic acid once hydrated, these preparations should be consumed immediately after mixing.

Vitamin C concentrations in fruits and vegetables vary widely. Since availability is not likely to be consistent in an emergency situation, this solution would not be applicable for acute cases. Oranges can provide 50–100 mg of vitamin C per serving, clearly a more-than-adequate source of the nutrient. Greens (such as collards or kale) would give about 20–30 mg per 1/2-cup serving. These foods would have to be supplied on a daily basis.

Prevention of Scurvy

Different approaches to prevent scurvy are possible in the short or long term. In the short term, prevention can be accomplished by (1) providing supplements of vitamin C, as described above for treatment of scurvy; (2) supplying vitamin C-fortified rations; (3) supplying vitamin C-containing foods as part of the ration package; or (4) ensuring access to local markets for acquisition of vitamin C-containing foods if they are available. It should also be recognized that breast milk is an excellent source of vitamin C (40 mg/L average; varies depending on vitamin C status of the mother), and efforts should be made to promote continued breast feeding of children. For situations in which the population is expected to be displaced for a long period, local food production might also be encouraged by providing seeds, tools, and appropriate training for establishing home or community gardens.

Vitamin C-Fortified Rations

If food commodities are adequately fortified with vitamin C and the vitamin is not destroyed during shipping, storage, or cooking, these rations should be adequate to prevent scurvy. The stability of vitamin C is discussed in Chapter 5. On the assumption that 6–10 mg per day would prevent scurvy, adequate intake of this minimum amount of vitamin C can be achieved from fortified rations by varying the amount of food provided. Regardless of the level of vitamin C in the ration, it is important to provide clear, simple instructions on appropriate cooking techniques to conserve vitamin C and on the desirability of consuming food as soon as possible following preparation.

To avoid the unnecessary cost of increased fortification for those populations that do not require it and the commonly experienced four- to six-month lag time between ordering commodities and their delivery in country, alternative approaches could be used.

Local Fortification

This approach, *which is already being used by the World Food Programme (WFP),* fortifies certain foods with additional vitamin C within the country or region in which particular relief programs are being implemented, only after a specific need has been identified. This approach requires both the availability of a specially formulated micronutrient mix that can be shipped rapidly to sites that require it and a local or regional processing capability. The committee was informed that specially fortified food can be obtained locally or regionally within a reasonably short period of time, although costs may be elevated when extraordinary procurement or shipping procedures are necessary.

Addition of Vitamin C-Containing Foods to Ration Packages

Another approach is to provide fresh or processed food sources of vitamin C as a component of the ration package. Examples might include locally purchased fresh fruit or vegetables or imported packaged items such as tomato paste, enriched powdered fruit drinks, and sour candies. The committee did not have access to information about the procurement and shipping costs of these items in different parts of the world, but it seems likely that they would be less than the cost of increasing the vitamin C content of *all* blended products if the items could be appropriately targeted to only those populations in need. Examples of the amounts of foods that would supply 10 mg of vitamin C (ascorbic acid) include 20 g of fresh orange (1/4 of a small orange), 30 ml of fresh lemon juice (bottled lemon juice is much lower in vitamin C), 25 g of tomato paste, or 2.5 g of powdered orange drink (USDA, 1997).

Ensuring Access to Market

When local sources of vitamin C are available in the marketplace, relief programs can be designed to take advantage of these foods. In particular, either foods can be procured locally by the program and distributed as described above, or the program can ensure that individual households have physical and economic access to the market. The latter approach can be facilitated by providing a sufficient amount of the basic staples to permit their exchange for vitamin C-containing foods without jeopardizing the adequacy of macro-nutrients provided by the relief package (Reed and Habicht, 1997).

Household Production of Vitamin C-Containing Foods

To reduce the burden on food distribution programs and decrease the dependence on donated foods, efforts should be made as soon as possible to facilitate local food production in situations where populations are likely to be displaced for long periods of time (i.e., more than one growing season). The extensive available literature on technical inputs required for promotion of home gardens can be adapted to increase the local availability of vitamin C-containing foods, at least during some parts of the year. These foods will also supply other needed nutrients.

Fortification of Title II Blended Commodities

Only a small proportion (~7 percent) of U.S.-supplied CSB and WSB is designated for emergency feeding programs in East African countries where scurvy has occurred. Although the United States supplied approximately 84 percent of all blended, fortified foods used worldwide (249,200 metric tons [MT]), 82 percent of U.S.-blended commodities went to Asia and to South and Central America. The majority of this 82 percent (75 percent) went to India for development feeding programs. Only 18 percent of U.S.-supplied CSB and WSB went to Africa, and roughly half of these went to general relief and to maternal and child health (MCH) programs rather than emergency programs. Of the 9–10 percent of CSB and WSB that was used for emergency feeding situations, only 70 percent would likely have been used in East Africa, where scurvy has been reported. Thus, fully 93 percent of the cost of adding more vitamin C to blended, fortified foods as a strategy for preventing scurvy is wasted. If a fixed dollar amount is assumed available for the purchase of food aid commodities, increasing the vitamin C content to 90 mg/100 g at an estimated increased cost of $6.33/MT would mean that approximately 425,800 fewer recipients could receive fortified, blended commodities as emergency food aid. This situation is not conducive to improving the nutrition and health status of refugees. Even if total food aid funding were increased, the same trade-off would exist in relation to the most effective use of increased funds.

Furthermore, the results of SUSTAIN's survey of five of the seven plants producing CSB or WSB raise serious questions about the capability of these manufacturers to meet specified fortification levels. Three of the five plants sampled were outside specifications almost 60 percent of the time, and levels fell below specifications more often than above. None of the plants sampled had a process capability (Cp) equal to or greater than 1.0. Given the pervasive problem of lack of uniformity of vitamin C content during the production of CSB and WSB, it would seem inappropriate to increase *any* micronutrient fortification of these commodities without better manufacturing controls.

The potential for fortified blends to prevent outbreaks of scurvy will depend on the extent of the losses of vitamin C that occur during transport, storage, and cooking. Information obtained from the pilot study indicates that vitamin C losses during shipment and storage are not a major concern. Conventionally fortified WSB shipped to Haiti indicated a small but significant loss of 13 percent, but vitamin C retention in the highly fortified WSB and conventionally fortified CSB was approximately 100 percent.

SUSTAIN's study indicates that losses of vitamin C during cooking may be a major limiting factor. The data for vitamin C losses during cooking are not conclusive because of a number of variables introduced, particularly the variability in vitamin C concentration of the starting blends (especially CSB) and the temperature or time of holding before cooked samples were frozen. The conclusions that are drawn relative to the concentration dependence of vitamin C retention are reasonable but not fully validated by the pilot studies. In addition, cooking times observed in the SUSTAIN study are not representative of emergency situations where fuel for cooking is frequently limiting.

Use of local food sources rich in vitamin C benefits the local economy and provides the additional nutrients in these foods; local foods can be obtained quickly to respond to the need for vitamin C in a timely way. Alternative approaches for the prevention of scurvy have to be explored where the availability of vitamin C-rich foods is low. Higher fortification of U.S.-provided blended foods is not the most efficient or cost-effective of these alternatives. In addition, although iron deficiency appears to be a much more widespread problem in emergency and development feeding situations, the use of higher levels of vitamin C fortification to enhance iron absorption is not a cost-effective method of improving iron status.

More cost-effective strategies would target populations at risk of vitamin C deficiency by providing vitamin C-containing foods as part of the emergency ration package; supplying a larger ration size of blended, fortified foods; ensuring access to local markets; or for long-term situations, encouraging local food production.

RECOMMENDATIONS

Major Recommendations

1. The level of vitamin C fortification of blended food aid commodities should NOT be increased to 90 mg/100 g but maintained at the current level of 40 mg/100 g. Based on the reported incidence of scurvy and the quantity of U.S.-supplied blended food commodities going to regions where scurvy has been reported, increasing the vitamin C fortification of all CSB and WSB is not cost-effective.

2. Strengthen health surveillance systems in refugee camps to monitor population risks of vitamin C deficiency and scurvy and to initiate a timely response. Risk factors for vitamin C deficiency and scurvy should be monitored at the community and/or camp level. Some of the risk factors that have been identified as potentially useful for such monitoring include: populations totally dependent on food aid (e.g., displaced and famine-affected populations [CDC, 1992]); duration of stay in a refugee camp (Toole, 1994); seasonality: dry season and inability to cultivate (Desenclos et al., 1989; Henry and Seaman, 1992); market failure, limited local supplies of fresh produce, or lack of resources to trade for other food sources (Magan et al., 1983; Toole, 1992); poor acceptance of donated foods, especially blended fortified foods, resulting from cultural preferences, (Mason et al., 1992; Toole, 1992); and difficult access for relief organizations because of war or remoteness (Mason et al., 1996). At the individual level, the risk factors include age and physiological status (young children, pregnant and lactating women, and the elderly have been found more susceptible).

3. Target identified populations at risk for scurvy with appropriate vitamin C interventions. There are several possible strategies to achieve increased vitamin C supplementation, (1) increased access to local foods and markets; (2) local fortification of commodities in the country or region where the emergency is occurring, as is currently practiced in some regions; and (3) use of vitamin C tablets if scurvy is already present. Alternatively, an increased total daily ration of conventionally-fortified, blended food would be appropriate in an emergency feeding situation and would increase the intake of other important nutrients such as energy, protein, and iron, as well as vitamin C. Another possibility might be for The U.S. Agency for International Development's (USAID's) Bureau of Humanitarian Response to investigate the logistics of managing two supplies of CSB and WSB, the conventionally-fortified blends, and a small proportion of highly-fortified blends that would only be targeted as part of the general ration to situations where the risk of vitamin C deficiency is high and continues for several months.

4. Improve the uniformity of blended food aid commodities by implementing specific product and process procedures. Delivery of vitamin and mineral fortification via food aid commodities to target populations depends on the manufacturing facilities' ability to comply with formulation and finished product specifications. To improve the uniformity of blended food, the following remedial initiatives are recommended:

• Formulation document—a formal reporting of the formulation and ingredients used to generate a particular product or blend.

• Product specifications—institute procedures for analytical quality control to monitor compliance with fortification levels defined by product specification. Inability of manufacturer to comply can result in loss of contract.

• Methods and Sampling Procedures—the list of all statistical process control procedures, all analytical procedures, test methods and the appropriate sampling protocols.

• Operating guide—a formal document that provides a blueprint for operating a process. It includes a process description for each step, a review of normal operating conditions, control actions (the set of steps necessary to maintain a quality operation), and a discussion of the impact of each process step on product quality.

• Control plan—a master document that keeps track of a plant's record keeping. It lists the specification or test to be performed, the source of the authority for the test, who is responsible for conducting the test, the test frequency, where the test is recorded, what action to take, and where to file or who must receive the report.

• HACCP (Hazards Analysis Critical Control Points) plan—a preventive system to identify key areas of process control to avoid food safety risks.

Measurements of improvement include analytical sampling and analysis of key fortification nutrients, regular audits of plant performance, maintenance of calibration records for all metering equipment, and maintenance of usage records for all vitamin and mineral premixes.

Research Recommendations

The committee has identified several areas in which additional research would be most helpful in alleviating potential vitamin C deficiencies and evaluating the appropriateness of any overall vitamin C fortification of U.S. commodities.

1. Research the epidemiology of vitamin C deficiencies. Ascertain the incidence of scurvy in displaced populations and analyze this according to the amount of blended, fortified foods received. The incidence of scurvy among those receiving blended foods at currently prescribed levels will permit assessment of the need to increase fortification or seek alternative approaches. Develop and validate predictors of populations at risk of vitamin C deficiency among refugees so as to institute local fortification

2. Research and develop means to increase consumption of local foods rich in vitamin C. This may also be achieved by purchasing such foods for refugees, but it may be done more cost-effectively by decreasing barriers to barter and trade in refugee camps.

3. Research and evaluate appropriate ration sizes of blended foods. More information is needed on the amounts of blended foods that are distributed to those at risk for scurvy in displaced populations. Currently, no good information is available on actual quantities distributed. This information may also indicate that much higher levels of fortification than are currently being considered are necessary for those at most risk because they could be receiving smaller rations.

4. Research and evaluate methods for campsite vitamin C fortification. This would be the most cost-effective approach to fortification because the need is rare and the cost of vitamin C is relatively high.

5. Research alternative forms of vitamin C available for fortification. The limited data available on cooking losses using the current ethyl cellulose-coated product indicates a need to develop other vitamin C products that are more stable to heating in dilute solutions.

References

ACC/SCN (United Nations Administrative Committee on Coordination/Subcommittee on Nutrition). 1996. Refugee nutrition information system. Update No. 2. November 11: 3–4.

ACC/SCN 1997. Update on the Nutrition Situation. SCN News 14 (July): 5–10.

Allen, L.H., and N. Ahluwalia. 1997. Improving iron status through diet. The Application of Knowledge Concerning Dietary Iron Bioavailability in Human Populations. Arlington, Va: OMNI.

Anderson, P., and P.T. Lukey. 1987. A biological role for ascorbate in the selective neutralization of extracellular phagocyte-derived oxidants. Ann. N.Y. Acad. Sci. 489:229–247.

Anderson, P., and A. Theron. 1979. Effects of ascorbate on leucoytes. Part III. In vitro and in vivo stimulation of abnormal neutrophil motility by ascorbate. S. Afr. Med. J. 56: 429–433.

Baker, E.M., R.E. Hodges, J. Hood, H.E. Sauberlich, S.C. March, and J.E. Canham. 1971. Metabolism of ^{14}C- and ^{3}H-labeled ascorbic acid in human scurvy. Am. J. Clin. Nutr. 24:444–454.

Beaton, G.H. 1995. Fortification of Foods for Refugee Feeding. Final Report to the Canadian International Development Agency and Technical Background Report: Derivations and Analysis. Willowdale, Ontario: GHB Consulting.

Calloway, D.H., S.P. Murphy, G.H. Beaton, D. Lein. 1993. Estimated vitamin intakes of toddlers: predicted prevalence of inadequacy in village populations in Egypt, Kenya, and Mexico. Am. J. Clin. Nutr. 58:376–384.

CDC (Centers for Disease Control and Prevention). 1989. Nutritional Status of Somali refugees—Eastern Ethiopia, September 1988—May 1989. MMWR 38(26):455–456, 461–463.

CDC 1992. Famine-affected, refugee, and displaced populations: Recommendations for public health issue. MMWR 41(13):14-16.

Cook, J.D., and E.R. Monson. 1977. Vitamin C, the common cold, and iron absorption. Am. J. Clin. Nutr. 30: 235–241

Cook, J.D., S.S.Watson, K.M. Simpson, D.A. Lipschitz, and B.S. Skikne. 1984. The effect of high ascorbic acid supplementation on body iron stores. Blood 64:712–726.

Dawson, W., and G.B. West. 1965. The influence of ascorbic acid on histamine metabolism in guinea pig. Br. J. Pharmacol. 24:725–734.

Desenclos, J.C. 1987. Relief food and vitamin C deficiency. Lancet (letter) Aug. 22:462–463.

Desenclos, J.C., A.M. Beiry, R. Podt, B. Farah, C. Segala, and A.M. Nabil. 1989. Epidemiological patterns of scurvy in Ethiopian refugees. Bull. WHO 67(3):309–316.

Erdman, J.W., Jr., and B.P. Klein. 1982. Harvesting, processing, and cooking influences on vitamin C in foods. *In Ascorbic Acid: Chemistry, Metabolism, and Uses.* P.A. Seib and B.M. Tolbert (eds.) Adv. in Chem. Ser. 200. Washington, D.C.:American Chemical Society.

Hallberg, L. 1981. The effect of vitamin C on the bioavailability of iron in food. (p. 49–61). *In Vitamin C: Ascorbic Acid.* J.N. Counsell and D.H. Horning (eds). Essex, England: Applied Science Publications.

Henry, C.J.K., and J. Seaman. 1992. The micronutrient fortification of refugee rations to prevent nutritional deficiencies in refugee diets. J. Refugee Studies 5(3/4):359.

Hodges, R.E., E.M. Baker, J. Hood, H.E. Sauberlich, and S.C. March. 1969. Experimental scurvy in man. Am. J. Clin. Nutr. 22:535–548.

Hodges, R.E., J. Hood, J.E. Canham, H.E. Sauberlich, and E.M. Baker. 1971. Clinical manifestations of ascorbic acid deficiency in man. Am. J. Clin. Nutr. 24:432–443.

Hornig, D.H. 1975. Metabolism of ascorbic acid. World Rev. Nutr. Diet. 23:225–258.

Hornig, D.H. and U. Moser. 1981. The safety of high vitamin C intakes in man. (p. 225–248). *In Vitamin C: Ascorbic Acid.* J.N. Counsell and D. Horning (eds.) Essex, England. Applied Science Publications.

IOM (Institute of Medicine). 1996. Vitamin C in Food Aid Commodities: Initial Review of a Pilot Program. Washington, D.C.: National Academy Press.

Irwin, M.I., and B.K. Hutchens. 1976. A conspectus of research on vitamin C requirements of man. J. Nutr. 106:823–879.

Leibovitz, B., and B.V. Siegel. 1978. Ascorbic acid, neutrophil function, and the immune response. Int. J. Vitamin Nutr. Res. 48:159–164.

Levenson, S.M., G. Manner, and E. Seifter. 1971. Aspects of the adverse effects of dysnutrition on wound healing. pp. 132–156. In *Progress in Human Nutrition, Vol. I.* S. Margen (ed.). Westport, Conn.: AVI Publishing.

Magan, A.M., M. Warsame, A. Oli-Salad and M.J. Toole. 1983. Outbreak of scurvy in Somali refugee camps. Disaster 7(2):94–97.

Mason, J., S. Gillespie, G. Clugston, and P. Greeves. 1992. Misconceptions on nutrition of refugees. Lancet (letter) 340:1354.

Mason, J., J. Wallace, J. Katona-Apte, and D. Alnwick. 1996. Nutrition and food aid: Methodologies. World Disasters Report. International Federation of Red Cross and Red Crescent Societies. Oxford, UK: Oxford University Press.

NRC (National Research Council). 1974. *Recommended Dietary Allowances,* eighth edition. Washington, D.C.: National Academy Press.

NRC (National Research Council). 1989. *Recommended Dietary Allowances,* tenth editon. Washington, D.C.: National Academy Press.

OMNI (Opportunities for Micronutrient Interventions). 1994. Micronutient Fortification and Enrichment of P.L. 480 Title II Commodities: Recommendations for Improvement. A Technical Review Paper. Arlington, Va.: OMNI.

Ranum, P., and F. Chomé (eds.). 1996. The Vitamin C Pilot Program: Monitoring, Evaluation, and Quality Control Component. Washington, D.C.: SUSTAIN.

Ranum, P. and F. Chomé (eds). 1997. Results Report on the Vitamin C Pilot Program. Washington, D.C.: SUSTAIN.

Reed, B.A. and J-P. Habicht. 1997. Sales of food aid as sign of distress, not excess. Lancet (in press).

Seaman, J., and J.P.W. Rivers. 1989. Scurvy and anemia in refugees. Lancet (letter) (May 27):1204.

Toole, M.J. 1992. Micronutrient deficiencies in refugees. Lancet (339):1214–1216.

Toole, M.J. 1994. Preventing micronutrient deficiency disease. Background document 2. ACC/SCN Workshop on Improvement of the Nutrition of Refugees and Displaced People in Africa. Machakos, Kenya.

UNHCR (United Nations High Commissioner on Refugees) 1989. Options to alleviate nutritional deficiency diseases in refugees. Discussion Paper. UNHCR. Technical Support Service.

USAID (United States Agency for International Development). 1990. Technical Review of Vitamin C and Iron Levels in P.L. 480 Title II Commodities, Arlington, Va.

USAID. 1996. FY 1996 Title II Emergency Program CSB/WSB Shipments. Arlington, Va.

USAID. 1997a. Metric Tonnage and Dollar Values (in $000's): Wheat Soy Blend. P.L. 480 Title II FY1996 Single Commodity Report.

USAID. 1997b. Metric Tonnage and Dollar Values (in $000's): Corn Soya Blend. P.L. 480 Title II FY 1996 Single Commodity Report.

USDA (United States Department of Agriculture). 1997. Nutrient Data Base for Standard Reference Release 11-1. [http://www.nal.usda.gov/fnic/foodcomp].

WHO (World Health Organization). 1993. Guidelines on Micronutrient Supplementation pp. 2–3, 8–12. Regional Office for Europe. Zagreb: Croatia.

Woodruff, C.W. 1975. Ascorbic acid—Scurvy. Prog. Food Nutr Sci. 1:493–506.

Appendix A

Legislative Language for Increased Vitamin C Fortification

SRpt 102-419 REPORT To accompany H.R. 5368
FOREIGN OPERATIONS, EXPORT FINANCING, AND RELATED PROGRAMS
APPROPRIATION BILL, 1993
Senate Appropriations
(COMREPORTS 09/23/92; 7770 lines)
Item Key: 2016

Special Typefaces Key:
  [[ ]] Text to be omitted   //   \\ Italic text
— — — — — — — — — — — — — — — —

INCREASE IN VITAMIN C FORTIFICATION

The Committee recommends that AID increase the fortification
level of vitamin C in AID export commodities from 40 to 100
milligrams per 100 gram ration, in the title II Public Law 480
program. The Committee believes that recent and continuing
scientific data has demonstrated that increased levels of vitamin C
are necessary to help decrease and eliminate health problems in
affected populations in recipient countries. Furthermore, increased
vitamin C fortification levels will help prevent diseases and health
problems, thus decreasing overall program and medical relief costs.

SRpt 103-142 REPORT To accompany H.R. 2295
FOREIGN OPERATIONS, EXPORT FINANCING, AND RELATED PROGRAMS
APPROPRIATION BILL, 1994
Senate Appropriations
(COMREPORTS 09/14/93; 7949 lines)
Item Key: 662

Special Typefaces Key:
  [[ ]] Text to be omitted   //   \\ Italic text
— — — — — — — — — — — — — — — —

VITAMIN C FORTIFICATION

Recipients of U.S. food aid in many nations suffer from
nutritional problems that could be alleviated, or in some cases
eliminated by the increased consumption of vitamin C. Recent studies
have shown, for example, that new mothers and infants can greatly
improve their health through consumption of this vitamin. One
effective means of increased vitamin C consumption is done by
increasing fortification levels of the commodities sent under title
II of the Public Law 480 Food Aid Program from the current level of
40 milligrams per 100 gram ration to 100 milligrams. In those cases
where no fortification exists, fortification should likewise be
started at 100 milligrams per 100 gram ration. The Committee notes
that improving the health of food aid recipients can reduce the need
for, and cost of, medical intervention at a later stage. The
Committee intends that AID expeditiously move to increase the
fortification levels of affected commodities.

****

HRpt 103-633 CONFERENCE REPORT To accompany H.R. 4426
MAKING APPROPRIATIONS FOR THE FOREIGN OPERATIONS, EXPORT FINANCING,
AND RELATED PROGRAMS FOR THE FISCAL YEAR ENDING SEPTEMBER 30, 1995
Conference Committee
(COMREPORTS 08/01/94; 3293 lines)
Item Key: 1707

Special Typefaces Key:
[[ ]] Text to be omitted   //   \\ Italic text
— — — — — — — — — — — — — — — —

103rd CONGRESS }   HOUSE OF REPRESENTATIVES   { Report
  2d Session }   { 103-633

MAKING APPROPRIATIONS FOR THE FOREIGN OPERATIONS, EXPORT FINANCING, AND RELATED PROGRAMS FOR THE FISCAL YEAR ENDING SEPTEMBER 30, 1995

August 1, 1994.—Ordered to be printed

Mr. OBEY, from the committee of conference, submitted the
following

CONFERENCE REPORT

[To accompany H.R. 4426]

The committee of conference on the disagreeing votes of the two
Houses on the amendments of the Senate to the bill (H.R. 4426)
"making appropriations for the Foreign Operations, Export Financing,
and Related Programs for the fiscal year ending September 30, 1995,"
having met, after full and free conference, have agreed to recommend
and do recommend to their respective Houses as follows:

VITAMIN C

The conferees believe that more accurate information is needed
regarding the fortification of food that is shipped overseas through
the Public Law 480 Food for Peace Program. The conferees therefore
request the Administrator of the Agency for International
Development to report to the Committees on Appropriations by
February 15, 1995 with an estimate of the cost of fortifying grains
shipped under the Public Law 480 program to 100 mg per 100 gram
ration and an assessment of whether or not the fortification of
grain is stable through the shipping process.

HRpt 104-143 REPORT To accompany H.R. 1868
 FOREIGN OPERATIONS, EXPORT FINANCING, AND RELATED PROGRAMS
APPROPRIATIONS BILL, 1996
House Appropriations
(COMREPORTS 06/15/95; 4457 lines)
Item Key: 453

Special Typefaces Key:
   [[ ]] Text to be omitted   //   \\ Italic text
— — — — — — — — — — — — — — — —

104th CONGRESS }   HOUSE OF REPRESENTATIVES   { Report
   1st Session }   { 104-143

FOREIGN OPERATIONS, EXPORT FINANCING, AND RELATED
PROGRAMS APPROPRIATIONS BILL, 1996

June 15, 1995.—Committed to the Committee of the Whole
House on the State of the Union and ordered to be printed

Mr. CALLAHAN, from the Committee on Appropriations,
submitted the following

R E P O R T

together with

MINORITY VIEWS

[To accompany H.R. 1868]

The Committee on Appropriations submits the following report in
explanation of the accompanying bill making appropriations for
Foreign Operations, Export Financing, and Related Programs, and for
sundry independent agencies and corporations for the fiscal year
ending September 30, 1996, and for other purposes.

VITAMIN C FORTIFICATION

Last year's report requested that AID increase vitamin C
fortification levels as part of the Public Law 480 Food Aid Program.
A report was submitted by AID on the cost of fortifying commodities
with vitamin C. While the study indicated that vitamin C may lose
stability over time and in the presence of moisture, the results
appear to be inconclusive as they affect Corn-Soy-Blend (CSB) and
Wheat-Soy-Blend (WSB), the principal commodities that are fortified.
Other studies have shown that new mothers and infants can greatly
improve their health through consumption of vitamin C.

The Committee recommends that AID perform a pilot program,
using up to $500,000 from the funds provided in this account,
involving the fortification of commodities with vitamin C, and
expects that the agency will report back on the results of that
pilot program by April 1, 1996.

SRpt 104-143 REPORT To accompany H.R. 1868
FOREIGN OPERATIONS, EXPORT FINANCING, AND RELATED PROGRAMS
APPROPRIATION BILL, 1996
Senate Appropriations
(COMREPORTS 09/14/95; 6006 lines)
Item Key: 740

Special Typefaces Key:
  [[ ]] Text to be omitted   //   \\ Italic text
— — — — — — — — — — — — — — — — —

104th CONGRESS }   SENATE   { Report
  1st Session }   { 104-143

FOREIGN OPERATIONS, EXPORT FINANCING, AND RELATED PROGRAMS
APPROPRIATION BILL, 1996

————

September 14 (legislative day, SEPTEMBER 5), 1995.–
Ordered to be printed

————

Mr. MCCONNELL, from the Committee on Appropriations,
submitted the following

REPORT

[To accompany H.R. 1868]

The Committee on Appropriations to which was referred the bill
(H.R. 1868), making appropriations for Foreign Assistance and
related programs for the fiscal year ending September 30, 1996, and
for other purposes, reports the same to the Senate with amendments
and recommends that the bill as amended do pass.

VITAMIN C FORTIFICATION

The Committee has included language for the last 3 years,
urging AID to increase vitamin C fortification in grains exported
through the Public Law 480 title II Food for Peace Program.
Recognizing AID's concerns regarding stability of the vitamin during
the shipping and cooking processes, the Committee has urged AID to
address and resolve these issues and remains concerned that AID has
yet to do so. Because the AID study to test the stability of vitamin
C in the shipping process was flawed, and an independent study
conducted with AID's approval proved that vitamin C is stable during
the cooking process, the Committee believes no further studies
should be undertaken. Thus, fortification levels of vitamin C should
be increased for the corn soy blend [CSB] and wheat soy blend [WSB]
exports. Studies show the health benefits of fortifying foods at the
RDA levels especially for new mothers and infants.

The Committee directs AID to perform a pilot program, as recommended in the House Committee report, utilizing up to $500,000 to increase the vitamin C fortification to the RDA level (90 mg per 1 gram ration for pregnant and lactating women) for CSB and WSB and other exported grains and cereals. AID will report back to the Committee by April 1, 1996, regarding the progress and any available results of the pilot program.

****

Appendix B

SUSTAIN Report Executive Summary

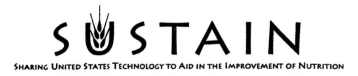

S U S T A I N

SHARING UNITED STATES TECHNOLOGY TO AID IN THE IMPROVEMENT OF NUTRITION

....

Results Report on the Vitamin C Pilot Program

**Submitted to the U.S. Agency for International Development for
Consideration by the Committee on International Nutrition of the
National Academy of Sciences**

Prepared by SUSTAIN
*(Sharing United States Technology to Aid in the
Improvement of Nutrition)*

Peter Ranum, Program Director
Françoise Chomé, Deputy Program Manager

September, 1997
Second Edition

....

SUSTAIN
1400 16TH STREET, N.W. · BOX 25 · WASHINGTON, D.C. 20036
202 328-5180 · FAX 202 328-5175 · SUSTAIN@SUSTAINTECH.ORG

EXECUTIVE SUMMARY

This report contains the results of the USAID Vitamin C Pilot Program for use by USAID in consultation with the National Academy of Sciences to determine appropriate vitamin C fortification levels in food commodities used in U.S. food aid programs.

The Vitamin C Pilot Program, initiated in March 1996, was designed to produce, provide, and evaluate food aid commodities with increased levels of vitamin C fortification. Using standard procedures, USAID's Food for Peace program procured two commodities for the pilot program. These commodities, corn soy blend (CSB) and wheat soy blend (WSB), were provided to Tanzania and Haiti at higher levels of vitamin C. SUSTAIN provided technical advice and monitored and evaluated the results of the program.

The report details the following monitoring results:

1. **The uniformity of vitamin C distribution in the products at five plant sites.** Vitamin C distribution at each plant site varied from plant to plant and within any given production run. The variability was particularly evident in CSB, which is produced by a continuous process. WSB, while produced in much more limited quantities, is processed by a batch system and showed more uniformity. The ability of the different plants to control the amount and variation of vitamin C added to the commodities was dependent on the type of processing equipment, plant design, and quality control procedures used in each plant.

2. **The stability of vitamin C from point of production to distribution of CSB shipped to India and of WSB shipped to Haiti.** The time involved for shipping, transport, and storage (nine months for Haiti and five months for India) resulted in very little loss of vitamin C. The WSB with the conventional level of added vitamin C that was sent to Haiti showed a small (13%) but significant ($P<.01$) loss of vitamin C. The WSB with the high level of added vitamin C and the CSB sent to India showed no significant ($P>.05$) change in vitamin C.[1]

3. **The variation of vitamin C distribution within bags after shipping and handling to Haiti and Tanzania.** Within-bag variation was tested after shipping and handling by sampling bags at two recipient sites from the top, middle, and bottom of the bag. There was variation among samples taken from the three bag locations but the variability was consistent throughout the bag, indicating that there was no systematic stratification or concentration of the vitamin within one part of the bag.

---

[1] The pilot CSB procurement sent to Tanzania could not be tested for vitamin C because the distribution of added micronutrients in this pilot procurement was not uniform. Therefore, it was deemed impractical for purposes of means comparisons; consequently, a procurement of conventional CSB shipped to India was substituted.

4. **The stability and presence of vitamin C after food preparation by recipients in a regular program in Haiti and an emergency program in Tanzania.** Retention of vitamin C added at conventional levels was between 17 and 32% in CSB gruel samples and was 27% in WSB gruel samples. Gruel samples containing 14% CSB or WSB are the most common foods prepared from these commodities, accounting for 62% of the 39 prepared food samples collected. CSB and WSB containing low levels (below 24 mg/100g) of vitamin C lose nearly all of the vitamin C during cooking. Conversely, the higher vitamin C levels allowed cooked food to retain some vitamin C at the time of consumption. The retention at high levels of added vitamin C was 56% in CSB gruel and 32% in WSB gruel. In the refugee camps in Tanzania, the next most common food made from CSB was "ugali," which contains 40% CSB. It showed an average vitamin C retention after cooking from 36 to 74% for ugali prepared with CSB containing high levels of vitamin C. In Haiti, the second most cooked dish made from WSB contained 80% WSB. This dish showed a mean vitamin C retention of 18% with WSB containing the conventional level of vitamin C and a mean retention of 33% with WSB containing the high level of vitamin C.

5. **A projection of the increased cost to the Food for Peace Program of increased levels of vitamin C.** The current price of the ethyl cellulose coated vitamin C used in conventional CSB and WSB (40mg/100g) is $9/kg or $3.69/MT of fortified CSB or WSB. The price of vitamin C fluctuates and is currently quite low compared to past years, when the cost was twice as high. If the ethyl cellulose coated vitamin C level of the commodities was increased from its present level of 40 mg/100g of commodity to 90 mg/100g, the cost would increase by $6.33/MT. Part of this cost increase can be attributed to having to use a more dilute vitamin premix, resulting in higher storage and shipping expenses.

These results are fully detailed in samples and analyses shown in the appendices.

The report also presents supplemental information requested by the Committee on International Nutrition of the National Academy of Sciences. Reports of scurvy outbreaks have been confined, except in rare occasions, to refugee populations in East Africa where refugees are largely dependent on food aid. SUSTAIN's literature search did not identify cases of scurvy that were attributed to food aid in regular development programs.

General rations containing inadequate vitamin C, combined with a lack of diversity of food sources, have been named as the primary factors for outbreaks of scurvy in displaced and famine-affected populations. Other characteristics are lack of ability to cultivate or trade for other food sources, remoteness and inaccessibility, cultural factors affecting food acceptance, and age and physiological status (pregnancy and lactation) of individuals in these situations. Many authors recommend 6 to 10 mg of vitamin C a day as a minimum requirement to prevent clinical manifestation of scurvy. The amount of vitamin C provided by CSB or WSB, containing 40 mg/100g of vitamin C at the point of consumption, when provided at a ration of 30 grams of CSB or WSB per day, would be 3.6 mg/day given a 30% cooking retention.

Until 1994, fortified cereal blends such as CSB and WSB were only occasionally provided in the general ration to refugees in East Africa when high prevalence of scurvy was determined. Most reported outbreaks of scurvy occurred before 1990. Fortified blended foods are now more routinely provided in emergency food aid program.

Use of vitamin C tablets was not found to be a practical method for preventing vitamin C deficiency in refugee populations.

Based on current production, increasing the level of vitamin C in all CSB and WSB produced to 90 mg/100g while keeping the current budget constant would reduce the tonnage produced by 4,662 metric tons and reduce the number of persons that could be fed a ration of 30 grams per day for a year by 425,797.

This report also includes information on alternative bagging, use of antioxidants, alternative forms of vitamin C, and iron fortification. Alternative forms of packaging are under consideration by the U.S. Department of Agriculture (USDA). USDA's primary interest in evaluating alternative packaging materials is to improve the strength of the bag rather than improving the micronutrient protection. Improved vitamin C protection does not appear necessary: this study showed relatively low levels of vitamin C degradation after shipping, handling, and storage.

A discussion of alternate forms of iron that might reduce the oxidation of vitamin C is also included in this report. However, this report also notes that further testing would be needed to determine the feasibility, acceptability, and cost of incorporating these other sources of iron into CSB and WSB.

The form of vitamin C currently used in CSB and WSB contains 97.5% ascorbic acid with a 2.5% ethyl cellulose coating. There are alternative forms of vitamin C now available with coatings of different types and thickness. These may provide better protection during food preparation than the current product, but no studies have been done to determine that. There are also other chemical forms of vitamin C with improved heat stability that are used in aquaculture, but none have been approved for human feeding.

I. OBJECTIVE

This activity provided technical information to the U.S. Agency for International Development (USAID) Vitamin C Pilot Program, which was designed to produce, provide, and evaluate food aid commodities that are fortified with increased levels of vitamin C. SUSTAIN specified the premix, recommended the pilot production quantity, and advised on field site selection. SUSTAIN also monitored and evaluated product quality, production costs, and vitamin C stability from the point of manufacture to the point of distribution and consumption. Two vitamin C fortified commodities used in the USAID Food for Peace Program were evaluated: corn soy blend (CSB) and wheat soy blend (WSB). This report presents results for use by USAID and the Committee on International Nutrition (CIN), Institute of Medicine of the National Academy of Sciences (NAS), to determine whether vitamin C levels in U.S. food aid commodities need to be increased.

II. BACKGROUND

Corn soy blend (CSB) and wheat soy blend (WSB) products are highly nutritious, low-cost, fortified foods that are used to deliver a wide array of macro- and micronutrients in the P.L. 480, Title II, Food for Peace Program. In fiscal year 1996 (October 1995 through September 1996), 238,300 metric tons (MT) of CSB and 11,310 MT of WSB were programmed for development activities and emergency activities such as refugee camp food distribution (USAID Annual Food Assistance Report, 1996). These blended cereal-based foods are partially precooked, which allows them to be easily incorporated into a number of different food preparations by recipients.

CSB and WSB are fortified with six essential minerals and eleven vitamins. This fortification accounts for 13% of the product cost. Like other P.L. 480 commodities, CSB and WSB are procured for USAID by the U.S. Department of Agriculture (USDA) Export Operations Division/Farm Service Agency. Currently there are seven different commercial companies approved by USDA to produce these commodities.

According to USDA guidelines, commodities must be produced in the United States under inspection by the USDA Grain Inspection, Packers and Stockyards Administration/Federal Grain Inspection Service (FGIS). An FGIS representative is present during commodity production and takes samples for analysis. Chemical and physical tests are run on these samples to determine compliance with specifications for the finished CSB/WSB. These routine tests include some nutritional analyses (protein, fat, moisture content, crude fiber), but they do not include tests for any of the added vitamins or minerals. Vitamin levels are not included in final product specifications. USDA composition specifications for CSB and WSB are contained in Appendix A.

CSB and WSB have vitamin C added in the ratio of 40 mg for every 100 g of commodity. The form of vitamin C currently used contains 97.5% ascorbic acid with a 2.5% ethyl cellulose coating. In September 1995, the U.S. Senate and House Appropriations Committees recommended that a pilot program be established to provide commodities with a 90 mg/100g fortification level (Foreign Operations, Export Financing, and Related Programs Appropriations Bill, 1996, S.Rpt. 104–143).

The operational component for the Vitamin C Pilot Program was implemented by the USAID Food for Peace Office in the Bureau of Humanitarian Response. It involved procuring, producing, and providing CSB with high and conventional levels of vitamin C to refugee camps in Tanzania and providing WSB with conventional and high levels of vitamin C to development programs in Haiti, using the usual program procedures for P.L. 480 Title II food aid.

The monitoring and evaluation component of the Vitamin C Pilot Program was conducted by SUSTAIN under a cooperative agreement with USAID. SUSTAIN, through the USAID Global Bureau's Office of Health and Nutrition in cooperation with the Program, Planning, and Evaluation office for the Bureau of Humanitarian Response (BHR), monitored the uniformity, stability and physical availability of vitamin C in the commodities from three selected country programs. In cooperation with the World Food Program (WFP), private voluntary organizations (PVOs), and USAID missions, SUSTAIN collected dry commodity samples in three countries. SUSTAIN also collected information about the local food preparation of the commodities and cooked samples in two countries, and determined vitamin C retention after cooking by testing samples of prepared food collected at recipient sites in these two countries.

The protocol for this activity was reviewed by an Advisory Panel of experts drawn from government, food relief agencies, and the food industry (Appendix B). These experts are knowledgeable in the fortification, stability, and testing of vitamins in these types of foods. This Advisory Panel met twice: once on April 18, 1996, to review the call forward request and sampling strategy, and again on May 17, 1996, to review the protocol. A statistical subgroup of the Advisory Panel, made up of statisticians and quality control experts of the food industry, advised on statistical matters and interpretation of the results (Appendix B). They met on May 3, 1996, to review the statistical plan of the study and to recommend the number of samples to be collected, and again on April 25, 1997, to discuss the statistical analysis of the results. Recommendations and suggestions from these meetings have been incorporated into this report. A protocol was designed and submitted to the Committee of International Nutrition (CIN) of the Institute of Medicine, National Academy of Science. Agreement on the protocol and recommendations by the CIN were presented to USAID in December 1996.

Appendix C

Letter from the United Nations World Food Programme

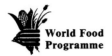

World Food Programme

Programa Mundial de Alimentos

Programme alimentaire mondial

بـرنامـج الأغذيـة العالمي

The Food Aid Organization of the United Nations System

10 June 1997

Dr. Mary Poos
Study Director, CIN
Food and Nutrition Board
Institute of Medicine
National Academy of Sciences
2101 Constitution Avenue, N.W.
Washington, D.C. 20418

Dear Dr. Poos:

Thank you for inviting me to comment on the task, "vitamin C in food aid commodities", before the the Institute of Medicine's Committee on International Nutrition of the National Academy of Sciences.

Currently there is increased attention focused on micronutrients, which is justified. The emphasis on vitamin C, however, is greater than the extent of its prevalence merits. Vitamin C deficiencies at present are reported from the Horn of Africa and from Nepal (Bhutanese refugees); this latter report is incorrect as the Bhutanese refugees receive micronutrient-fortified blended food as well as fresh vegetables. The report from the Horn, largely Somali refugees, is of small seasonal outbreaks which are effectively controlled with blended food distribution. Vitamin C deficiency occurs infrequently and only in particular situations, and when it is identified, interventions are introduced to correct it.

In the large majority of refugee situations and other distribution programmes where blended foods are used, there are no indications of Vitamin C deficiency. Considering the special circumstances of Vitamin C deficiency, WFP does not consider it justified to increase the Vitamin C content of the entire production of blended foods to meet some occasional instances of deficiency. Fortification with Vitamin C is very expensive, it accounts for about one third of the cost of the vitamin premix added to blended foods. The adoption of higher vitamin C levels will, therefore, result in significant price increases for blended foods.

The Committee should keep in mind that while the need for food aid is increasing, the quantity available is decreasing. In 1996 global food aid deliveries were 24 percent less than in 1995, and 55 percent less than in 1993. The 7.5 million tons delivered in 1996 were well below the annual target of 10 million tons established by the World Food Conference in 1974.

Forty-four percent of global food aid deliveries were financed by the United States last year, of which a little over seven percent (247,127 metric tons) were blended foods, the commodity under consideration by your committee. Note, however, that this is 84 percent of the total (294,554 mt) blended food used world wide. Most of the US provided blended food goes to Asia, in fact 90 percent of it (195,415 mt) to India. As far as I know, there are no reports of Vitamin C deficiency where most of the US-provided blended food is distributed.

In the final conclusion it all comes down to cost. While higher levels of fortification are desirable, a greater volume of food is even more critically needed. Increased fortification will raise costs while reducing the total quantity of food available for humanitarian assistance. In the case of India, for example, higher per metric ton costs will result in reduced quantities of food being available, leading to fewer children receiving supplementary feeding.

There are some 600 million food insecure people in the world. Any action that will further reduce the potential quantity of food available for them is not advisable. When there is a need for additional vitamin C, there are mechanisms already in existence to provide it.

Sincerely yours,

Judit Katona - Apte

Judit Katona-Apte, Dr.P.H.
Senior Programme Officer

Appendix D

Biographical Sketches

Lindsay H. Allen, Ph.D., R.D., (Chair), is professor of nutrition at the University of California at Davis. She received the 1997 Kellogg International Nutrition Prize and was the first President of the Society for International Nutrition Research. Dr. Allen is a member of IOM's Food and Nutrition Board and of their Standing Committee on the Scientific Evaluation of Dietary Reference Intakes, and the U.S. Committee of the International Union of Nutritional Sciences. She is associate editor for The Journal of Nutrition where she is responsible for Community and International Nutrition, and is on the Board of Directors for the International Nutrition Foundation for Developing Countries. Dr. Allen's expertise is in the determination of the causes and consequences of micronutrient deficiencies, and approaches for their prevention.

Kenneth H. Brown, M.D., is professor of nutrition and director of the Program of International Nutrition at the University of California at Davis. He currently serves as a member of the editorial board for the *European Journal of Clinical Nutrition* and as an assistant editor for the *American Journal of Clinical Nutrition*. From 1993 until 1996, Dr. Brown was the president of the Society for International Nutrition Research. Dr. Brown's research has focused on nutritional intervention for diarrheal diseases in malnourished children, and in 1995 he was awarded the International Nutrition Research Prize by the Society for International Nutrition Research.

Gus D. Coccodrilli, Ph.D., is vice president of Worldwide Scientific Relations, Nutrition, and External Technology for Kraft Foods Inc. As a member of the American Society of Nutritional Sciences, he served on the ASNS/ASCN Joint Membership Committee and chaired the Industry Liaison Committee. He also belongs to American Men and Women in Science and the

Institute of Food Technologists. Dr. Coccodrilli is a member of the Board of Trustees for the International Life Sciences Institute and serves as an advisor to the Monell Chemical Senses Center.

Jean-Pierre Habicht, M.D., Ph.D., is professor of nutritional epidemiology in the Division of Nutrition Sciences at Cornell University. His other professional experience includes special assistant to the director of the Division of Health Examination Statistics at the National Center for Health Statistics, World Health Organization (WHO), medical officer at the Instituto de Nutricion de Centro America y Panama, and professor of maternal and child health at the University of San Carlos in Guatemala. Currently, Dr. Habicht serves as an adviser to United Nations and government health and nutrition agencies. He is a member of the Expert Advisory Panel on Nutrition, WHO, and has been a member of the IOM's Food and Nutrition Board and the UN Advisory Group on Nutrition. He has consulted to the United Nations' World Food Programme and is involved in research with the United Nations High Commission for Refugees about the adequacy of food rations in refugee camps.

Barbara P. Klein, Ph.D., is professor of foods and nutrition in the Department of Food Science and Human Nutrition and Division of Nutritional Sciences in the College of Agricultural, Consumer, and Environmental Sciences at the University of Illinois at Urbana-Champaign. She served as head of the Department of Foods and Nutrition from 1985 until 1990 and chaired the College Promotions and Tenure Committee. Her research deals with the nutrient content of food as it is consumed after preparation and/or processing. Dr. Klein is editor of two books (including *Methods of Vitamin Assay*) and author of seven book chapters and many journal articles and presentations. Dr. Klein received the Borden Award for Foods Research in 1988 and the Paul A. Funk Award for Excellence from her College in 1997; she was elected a fellow in the Institute of Food Technologists in 1994. She serves as an elected member of the Executive Committee of the Institute of Food Technologists and was associate scientific editor of the *Journal of Food Science*.

George P. McCabe, Ph.D., is professor of statistics and head of the Statistical Consulting Service at Purdue University. He is also a fellow of the American Statistical Association. He presently serves as statistical design consultant for the journal *Augmentative and Alternative Communication* and associate editor for *Computational and Data Statistics*. In 1995, he served as guest researcher in the Statistical Engineering Division of the Computing and Applied Mathematics Laboratory at the National Institute of Standards and Technology. Previously, he was a guest researcher at the Commonwealth Scientific and Industrial Organization (CSIRO) in Melbourne, Australia, and at the University of Berne in Switzerland. He is coauthor of the textbook,

Introduction to the Practice of Statistics. Dr. McCabe's research interests include applied statistics, mathematical statistics, statistical computing, and statistics and the law. Dr. McCabe received his B.S. degree in mathematics from Providence College, and his Ph.D. in mathematical statistics from Columbia University

Beatrice L. Rogers, Ph.D., is dean for academic affairs and professor of economics and food policy at the Tufts University School of Nutrition Science and Policy. She is an economist specializing in food policy. She has done research on household income, prices, and other determinants of food consumption and household food security in numerous countries, including the United States, Pakistan, Honduras, the Dominican Republic, and Mali. She has also done research on the dynamics of intrahousehold resource allocation, focusing on income sources, use of time of household members, and how these factors affect food consumption, health, and nutritional status. Dr. Rogers has designed and implemented national household income, expenditure, and consumption surveys in several countries. She has worked on evaluations of the uses of food aid, most recently conducting a formal cost-effectiveness analysis of alternative food aid programs in Honduras. She is actively involved in the development of educational programs in the field of public nutrition, studying the determinants of nutrition in populations, and focusing especially on how the nutritional well-being of populations is affected by public policies outside the health or nutrition sector.

Marie Ruel, Ph.D., is currently a research fellow at the International Food Policy Research Institute (IFPRI) in Washington. She is in charge of a multicountry research program to analyze the food security and nutrition implications of rapid urbanization in developing countries. She also conducts research on strategies to alleviate micronutrient deficiencies. Before joining IFPRI in 1996, she was head of the Human Nutrition Division at the Institute of Nutrition of Central America and Panama (INCAP) in Guatemala. She has a Ph.D. in international nutrition from Cornell University.